Non-Surgical Thread Procedures

AF382680

Nancy M. Kim

Non-Surgical Thread Procedures

The Future of Aesthetic Medicine

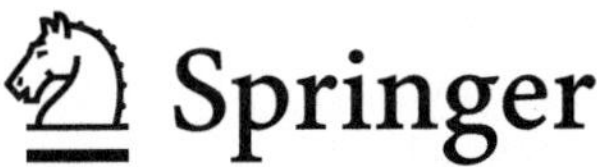

Nancy M. Kim
Adagio Aesthetic Medicine and
Thread Lift Center
Los Angeles, CA, USA

ISBN 978-3-031-36470-9   ISBN 978-3-031-36468-6   (eBook)
https://doi.org/10.1007/978-3-031-36468-6

© The Editor(s) (if applicable) and The Author(s), under exclusive license to Springer Nature Switzerland AG 2023
This work is subject to copyright. All rights are solely and exclusively licensed by the Publisher, whether the whole or part of the material is concerned, specifically the rights of translation, reprinting, reuse of illustrations, recitation, broadcasting, reproduction on microfilms or in any other physical way, and transmission or information storage and retrieval, electronic adaptation, computer software, or by similar or dissimilar methodology now known or hereafter developed.
The use of general descriptive names, registered names, trademarks, service marks, etc. in this publication does not imply, even in the absence of a specific statement, that such names are exempt from the relevant protective laws and regulations and therefore free for general use.
The publisher, the authors, and the editors are safe to assume that the advice and information in this book are believed to be true and accurate at the date of publication. Neither the publisher nor the authors or the editors give a warranty, expressed or implied, with respect to the material contained herein or for any errors or omissions that may have been made. The publisher remains neutral with regard to jurisdictional claims in published maps and institutional affiliations.

This Springer imprint is published by the registered company Springer Nature Switzerland AG
The registered company address is: Gewerbestrasse 11, 6330 Cham, Switzerland

Preface

Although thread procedures have been used for many years in other countries such as South Korea, in the USA, it is a relatively new procedure. Only in the last few years has thread procedures become more widely available and recognized in the USA. Thread procedures are still in the infancy of its development as a major treatment utilized by practitioners compared to botulinum toxins, fillers, and lasers. This is partially because PDO threads were introduced in the US market only about 6 years ago. Thread procedures also require training and skill that is more complex than procedures such as botulinum toxin or fillers. This book was written to serve as a primer for practitioners including physicians and nurses who are interested in learning how to perform thread procedures. Thus far, there have only been books either written by authors from other countries or translated into English from other languages. Most of the books are either outdated or partially irrelevant to the current thread market in the USA. This is the first book originally written in the English language and written by an author practicing currently in the USA. It is directed towards practitioners who are new to threads as well as those with experience. Since thread procedures offer and benefit from creative and wide variations, it is always useful to get new ideas from practitioners. This book is certainly not meant to be a substitute for hands-on training. For thread procedures in particular, it is paramount that the procedures are first attempted under direct hands-on guidance of an experienced practitioner. Links to instructional videos (Chap. 33) are also included to provide an opportunity to observe and study the thread procedure prior to obtaining hands-on training.

I thank my colleagues Dr. Vincent Wong and Dr. Michelle Reyes who helped make this book possible. I am grateful to have supportive fellow pioneers in this journey exploring the power of thread procedures. I would also like to thank all my patients who agreed to allow their photos and videos to be included in the textbook for their trust in me. Finally, I thank my dear friends and family who provided support and encouragement.

Los Angeles, CA, USA   Nancy M. Kim

Contents

Chapter 1
The History of Threads

Threads or barbed suture were first utilized for cosmetic procedures to lift facial tissue as early as the 1990s by Sulamanidze and colleagues (2002). These sutures named Aptos threads were non-absorbable and made of polypropylene in contrast to current threads which are absorbable and primarily made of polydioxanone. There were many reports of complications due to the Aptos threads, including extrusion, migration, infection, scarring that occurred even years after the procedure. Their popularity waned and the threads at that time did not gain FDA approval.

Subsequently another suture called Contour Threads, which were again non-absorbable polypropylene with barbs, did achieve FDA approval in 2004. However, these were shortly thereafter reported to have a high rate of complications including infection, extrusion, severe pain, swelling and recurrent laxity. The FDA approval was revoked only 3 years later.

Due to the high rate of complications with non-absorbable suture material, absorbable sutures emerged as the safer albeit temporary option. It has since established a stable and growing presence in the US market. Absorbable PDO threads were first introduced in the United States in 2016 after their FDA approval. They have been in use for a much longer time in other countries, however and is established as a popular technique with extensive product variations. For example, in South Korea, absorbable PDO threads for aesthetic purposes were first introduced in 2011 and there are more than 20 thread manufacturers or distributors while in the USA there are only six thread companies that primarily market threads. Threads in the USA however are beginning to grow in popularity among patients in recent years. Social Media has helped fuel its growing recognition as an effective treatment. For example, thread lift for the eyebrows has become desirable among the younger generation and is referred to by them as the "fox eyes" thread lift.

© The Author(s), under exclusive license to Springer Nature
Switzerland AG 2023
N. M. Kim, *Non-Surgical Thread Procedures*,
https://doi.org/10.1007/978-3-031-36468-6_1

Reference

Sulamanidze MA, et al. Removal of facial soft tissue ptosis with special threads. Dermatol Surg. 2002;28:367–71.

Chapter 2
Importance of Thread Procedures in the Current Landscape of Cosmetic Procedures

Thread procedures are positioned to become revolutionary in the aesthetic field. Thread procedures with the use of barbed or cogged sutures have the unique ability to reposition skin as well as induce significant collagenesis. Traditional surgical facelifts do not provide this dual benefit. In addition, thread procedures are minimally invasive therefore not requiring surgery nor general anesthesia. The recovery compared to that after surgery is much less taxing on the patient with only mild-moderate swelling resolving after 1 week, rare instances of bruising, and ability to return to work and engage in daily activities the same or next day. Only local anesthesia rather than general anesthesia is required decreasing the overall risk of adverse outcomes and allowing patients of any age and co-morbid conditions to still be eligible. And yet it can approach results that can be obtained with traditional surgical face lifts with completely natural looking results. There is little risk of significant change in one's characteristic features, no scarring, and true cellular anti-aging. In contrast to traditional surgical face lifts, the skin quality is improved at the histological level with augmentation of collagen production induced by the threads which would not necessarily occur after a surgical facelift. In addition, thread procedures are accessible to a broader range of age and affluence while surgical face lifts given the much higher cost, down time, and risk are limited to a smaller group of patients.

Apart from the surgical options, in the field of aesthetic medicine, prior to threads there have been ways to either plump up skin with hyaluronic acid fillers or increase collagen via non-invasive technologies but not directly reposition skin. The other very common modality, botulinum toxin neuromodulators, suppress muscle activity to diminish the appearance of fine lines. Neuromodulators may alter positioning of skin slightly by affecting muscle activity but do not directly change the position of the skin relative to the muscle layer nor do they induce collagenesis. Modalities like PRP, other bio-stimulatory injections and non-invasive technologies are designed to improve the collagen composition and quality of the skin, however, the improvement is usually mild-moderate. In addition, these do not significantly alter the position of

© The Author(s), under exclusive license to Springer Nature Switzerland AG 2023
N. M. Kim, *Non-Surgical Thread Procedures*, https://doi.org/10.1007/978-3-031-36468-6_2

the skin in relation to the muscular layer directly to a significant degree, and thus do not improve sagging directly. PDO threads and threads of other composition are revolutionary in this sense. When designed with barbs, cogs or other modifications, threads can significantly re-position the skin in relation to the overlying muscle layer as well as significantly change the composition of the skin regarding increased collagen potentially more than any other modality.

Despite the inherent value of the procedures, some factors have stymied its growth in the aesthetic field. These factors have included resistance by the cosmetic surgical community and the higher level of skill required to perform the procedure successfully. The technique of using PDO threads especially the barbed threads do require practice and courage to develop a comfortable level of skill. The procedure requires more practice as it is less intuitive and simple compared to botulinum toxin or filler injections which require only use of a small needle and syringe. The advanced manual skill needed and the variety of threads to choose among require significant experience and understanding to obtain good results. This book will hopefully help clinicians develop a better understanding of threads and techniques so that the true potential of threads to improve patient's aesthetic needs for anti-aging can be fully blossomed. It would be a shame to deny patients the extreme benefit that can be attained by thread procedures. Threads provide significant notice-able improvement in ways that are not achievable with other modalities including surgical face lifts, botulinum toxins, fillers, and non-invasive technologies. It is an invaluable armament in the fight against the aging process. It is a revolutionary modality that must be spread rather than stymied by any unwarranted resistance or lack of commitment and diligence to develop proper skill.

Chapter 3
Research Supporting the Efficacy of Thread Procedures

Thread procedures are relatively new in the aesthetic field and thus, there is much questioning of whether they are effective or worth the cost and effort. There is also naturally resistance among the plastic surgery community since thread procedures may ultimately replace the traditional surgical facelift. Patients who get thread procedures done on a regular basis may ultimately be able to prevent aging and obviate a surgical face lift in the future. A review of literature indeed reveals effectiveness of thread procedures, high patient satisfaction levels, and low incidence of complications based on clinical trials. In addition, an accurate average cost reported is significantly lower than surgery, solidifying the inherent value of threads in the fight against aesthetic aging.

Resistance to acceptance of thread procedures as a viable option seems unreasonable or founded on false information. There has, in fact, been objective evidence of the effectiveness of thread lift procedures provided by clinical studies. One study looking at 2 years outcome after thread lifting showed that there was significant long-lasting effects and a high degree of patient satisfaction. Skin lifting was found to be between 3 and 10 mm with a very low incidence rate of complications at 4.8% (Ali 2018). Another study of neck rejuvenation with thread lift showed statistically significant improvement with only minor complications including bruising and edema that lasted for only 72 h and no other complications thereafter (Arora and Arora 2019). A review of 59 articles about thread lifting was done to investigate the safety and adverse effects of the procedure. The study showed that most side effects associated with threads were self-resolving and any more serious cases subsided with treatment. Serious adverse effects, however, were rare (Pham et al. 2021). A study doing a perspective chart review of a total of 151 patients who underwent various thread lift procedures including for the mandible, mid face, neck, and eyebrow showed a very high level of satisfaction for patients of 89% 6 months after the procedure. Satisfaction level by the surgeon was 95%. What was also interesting about the study was that the level of satisfaction was found to increase over time from the first week after the procedure to the sixth month after the

© The Author(s), under exclusive license to Springer Nature Switzerland AG 2023

N. M. Kim, *Non-Surgical Thread Procedures*,
https://doi.org/10.1007/978-3-031-36468-6_3

procedure (Rezaee Khiabanloo et al. 2019). This is important to keep in mind when you enter the practice of doing thread lifts. It is important to reassure the patient that the results are optimal with some passage of time of a few weeks to months.

Despite the plethora of articles showing high levels of patient satisfaction there remains resistance among the cosmetic surgical community as this is a relatively new treatment modality and potentially a threat to the value of surgical facelifts. However, one must keep in mind that studies consistently show that patient satisfaction is very high and complication rates are very low and relatively less serious compared to surgical risk. One must be careful to not be misled and instead aim to steadfastly hold to truthful facts and experience. For example, in an article that ultimately concluded that thread lift procedures were not useful for most patients, the study demonstrated that patients had a very high level of satisfaction—rating it 8–9 out of 10 for all patients in the study (Dario Bertossi et al. 2019). The authors conclusion that the procedure was not worthy was, in fact, based only on erroneous information. They compared the cost of thread lift to traditional surgical facelift and stated that it was 40% of the cost of a traditional facelift, however, their quotation of the cost of PDO thread lift as $4000 is mistaken. Most PDO thread lifts in the area they referred to (the mandibular line or malar area) averages in the US between $500 and $800 which is only 10% of the cost of a traditional surgical facelift (Francesco and Bernardini 2019). Thus, the value of this procedure is hard to be refuted given that the objective results of the study was, in fact, favorable in terms of patient satisfaction. Even in this one article (Dario Bertossi et al. 2019) that concluded that PDO thread lifts were not to be recommended for most patients over surgical face lift, the conclusion could only be made based on a false premise that the cost of a thread lift was high relative to its longevity. The merits of the procedure itself could not be refuted by the data obtained in their study.

References

Ali YH. Two years' outcome of thread lifting with absorbable barbed PDO threads: innovative score for objective and subjective assessment. J Cosm Laser Ther. 2018;10(1):41–9.

Arora G, Arora S. Neck rejuvenation with thread lift. J Cutan Aesthet Surg. 2019;12(3):196–200.

Dario Bertossi M, et al. Effectiveness, longevity, and complications of facelift by barbed suture insertion. Aesthet Surg J. 2019;39(3):241–7.

Francesco P, Bernardini M. Is there a role for a noninvasive alternative to face and neck lifting? The polydioxanone thread lift. Aesthet Surg J. 2019;39(8):NP362–3.

Pham CTM, Chu SD, Foulad DPM, Mesinkovska NAMP. Safety profile of thread lifts on the face and neck: an evidence-based systematic review. Dermatol Surg. 2021;47(11):1460–5.

Rezaee Khiabanloo S, et al. Innovative techniques for thread lifting of face and neck. J Cosmet Dermatol. 2019;18:1846–55.

Chapter 4
Biochemical and Physical Properties of Threads

Threads for esthetic procedures originate from materials created for other uses including sutures for surgery. The most used type or material is PDO or polydioxanone. Polydioxanone is a colorless, crystalline polymer that is biosynthetic and biodegradable. It was developed in 1982 for use as surgical sutures but is now also used in vascular grafts and even as scaffolding for cultivation of human organs and tissues. Polydioxanone is degraded by hydrolysis and its end products are mainly excreted in the urine with the remainder exhaled as CO_2 or eliminated by the digestive system (Kariduraganavar et al. 2014). It is well tolerated by the body and is resistant to infection (Weitzel and Taylor 2005).

The molecules used to form threads stimulate fibroblasts to create collagen. Similar to how oysters will build a nacre around a foreign body and create a beautiful pearl, these threads stimulate the body to grow collagen into the skin thereby imparting improved skin quality. The result is more firm, taut skin, brighter skin tone, decreased pore size, decrease in abnormal pigmentation, and decreased acne. The change is most visible after 1–2 months. The improvement in skin quality is significant enough to be noticeable to the patient as well as to unbiased relations who have no knowledge that any procedure was performed. This is an advantage over surgical face lift which does not biologically change the skin even though it may appear smoother due to surgical removal of excess skin and repositioning of remaining skin. With surgery, skin is of the same composition with no added collagen. With thread procedures, the skin is noticeably thicker and tauter due to increase in collagen. The result will of course depend on the age and prior condition of the skin but there is always improvement that is noticeable as long as enough threads are placed. Some threads stimulate more collagen than others because of more presence of the material. For example, if it is a polydioxanone mesh thread then there will be more polydioxanone. The thread may be thicker or be a combination of multiple thin threads so that there is more polydioxanone to trigger more collagen building by the skin.

© The Author(s), under exclusive license to Springer Nature Switzerland AG 2023
N. M. Kim, *Non-Surgical Thread Procedures*, https://doi.org/10.1007/978-3-031-36468-6_4

Threads are sutures that are of different shapes, sizes, and designs. In surgery, some designs of the suture surface allow for tissue approximation without needing to tie knots as necessary with other surgical suture technique. These designs involve some type of alteration of the smooth surface of the suture so that instead of smoothly passing in and out through tissue, the suture will "snag," or grab hold when being moved through tissue. If the design of the surface of the suture is such that the "snag" is strong enough to cause the suture to be unable to be moved unless significant power is applied, the suture can be used to pull together different areas of tissues and affix them in place relative to each other. For example, an open wound can be closed with barbed sutures without tying knots. A study was done with dogs showing that a wound closed with barbed sutures can hold against disturbance and tension created by movement by the dog equally as well as a wound closed with multiple sutures held with knots (Jeffrey and Leung 2006). An analogy can be helpful to understand this phenomenon when you consider two pieces of wood held together by a screw versus the same pieces held together by smooth nails. It is more difficult to pull apart objects held by screws than nails. In the face that is sagging, there are not open wounds but there are gaps in the tissue where loss of fat, collagen, fibers have been lost and the tissues are not in the positions of the more youthful state. The barbed threads can close the gaps physically and then induce contraction of overlying excess skin by collagen stimulation.

Clinically, effects after the placement of threads include improved skin elasticity with a smaller facial contour and brightening of the complexion. This was seen in a study done to determine the histologic changes that are responsible for the aesthetic results. The study placed threads into a specific variety of pig skin that resembled the structure of human skin. Forty-eight weeks after the threads were inserted a histological analysis was performed. It showed that surrounding the threads there was neocollagenesis, fat reduction, tissue contraction, a fibrous merging effect, and an improved vascular environment (Yoon 2019). These histologic changes are indeed explanatory and consistent with what is apparent upon viewing the patient.

References

Jeffrey C, Leung GL. Barbed, bi-directional surgical sutures. In: Anand JKSC, editor. Medical textiles and biomaterials for healthcare. New Delhi: Woodhead Publishing; 2006. p. 395–403.

Kariduraganavar MY, Kittur AA, Kamble RR. Polymer synthesis and processing. In: Kumbar SG, Laurencin CT, Deng M, editors. Natural and synthetic biomedical polymers. Amsterdam: Elsevier; 2014. p. 1–31.

Weitzel S, Taylor S. Suturing technique and other closure materials. In: Robinson JK, editor. Surgery of the skin. St. Loius, MO: Mosby; 2005. p. 225–44.

Yoon JH. Tissue changes over time after polydioxanone thread insertion: an animal study with pigs. J Cosmet Dermatol. 2019;18(3):885–91.

Chapter 5
Threads Counter the Anatomy of Aging

While different people may age differently and at variable rates, there are characteristic changes that occur in many people during the aging process. These changes may include among others, descent of the eyebrows and eyelids, tear trough formation, flattening of the cheeks, deepening of nasolabial folds, and jowls formation. Figure 5.1 illustrates what we see in the aged face compared to the youthful face. The underlying cause of these changes is felt to be multifactorial and include volume loss, ligament attenuation, fat atrophy, loss of skin elasticity, bone loss, muscular changes, and gravitational forces (Wulc et al. 2012). Except for bone loss, threads can be useful to counteract all these forces of aging. For example, specifically addressing the changes shown in Fig. 5.1, the eyebrows and eyelid can be lifted with barbed threads and the brow bone flattening remedied with volumizing mesh threads. The tear trough can be volumized and skin laxity combatted with mesh threads. The nose tip and bridge can be lifted with nose threads. The nasolabial fold, marionette lines, and chin can be volumized with mesh threads. The neck can be lifted with barbed threads. Finally, the cheeks and jowls can be lifted with barbed threads.

With regard specifically to the cheeks and jowls, in addition to descent inferiorly of tissues, there is also a forward collapse. The bony structures shrink, ligaments become more relaxed, fat atrophies and migrates, and skin becomes less elastic. All these factors cause involution of the face or prolapse anteriorly in addition to inferiorly. It is not just that the cheek moves downward from above to accumulate over the nasolabial fold but also that it moves from lateral to medial. Similarly, the jowls form not only due to descent from above but also from tissue prolapsing forward anteriorly. One can demonstrate this as was done in an article by Allan E. Wulc et al. where they showed that tissues when allowed to move back laterally towards the borders of the face by placing the face supine, many of the features of the aged face were improved. I have been able to confirm this as well as shown in Fig. 5.2. When the patient is upright as shown in the first image in Fig. 5.2, the cheek, jowls, and nasolabial fold falls forward. It is not necessary to have the patient

© The Author(s), under exclusive license to Springer Nature
Switzerland AG 2023
N. M. Kim, *Non-Surgical Thread Procedures*,
https://doi.org/10.1007/978-3-031-36468-6_5

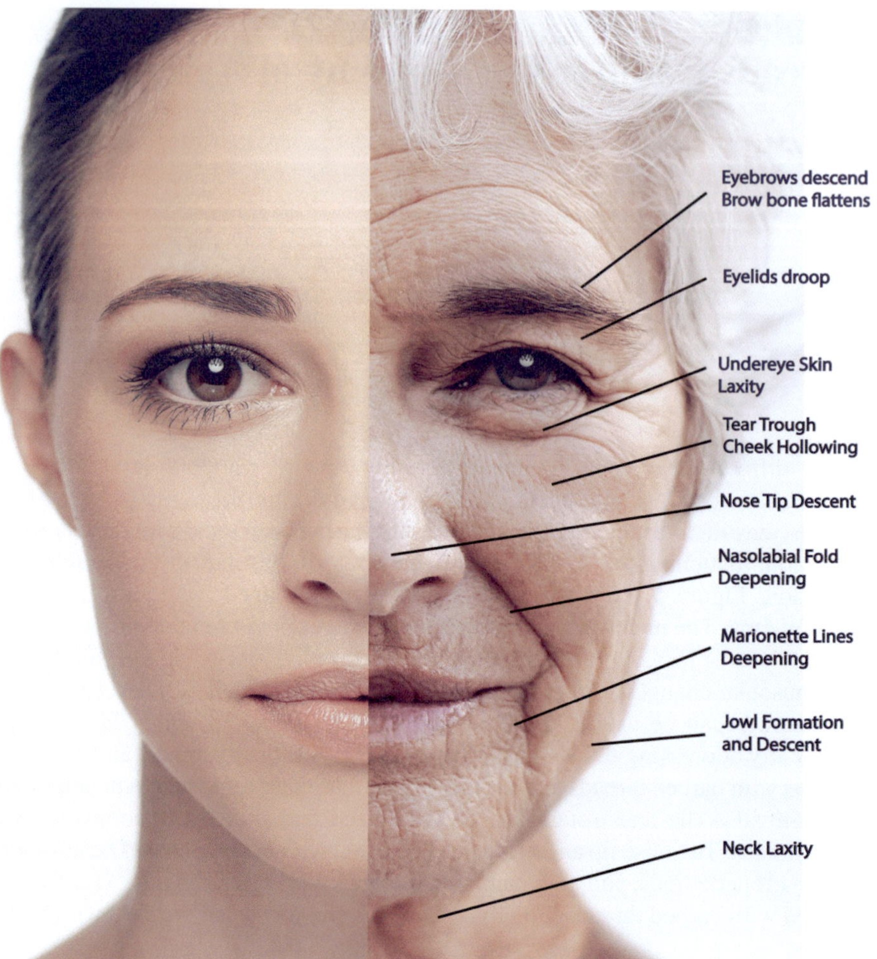

Fig. 5.1 Illustration of the aged face versus the youthful face with markers of changes that occur with aging

be upside down to improve the facial features but in fact even just being positioned supine as shown in the second image in Fig. 5.2 and allowing the tissues to drape over the skeletal structure of the face peripherally towards the hairline and posterior mandible restores a more youthful appearance. Thus, one can postulate that there becomes a wider separation of tissues from the outer borders of the face to the central region leading to accumulation of tissues centrally as well as inferiorly. This separation is created partially by ligament laxity, skin laxity, and fat atrophy leaving pockets of emptied tissue.

This separation of tissues can be addressed using threads. One can consider the threads as being utilized to approximate the tissues that have been displaced

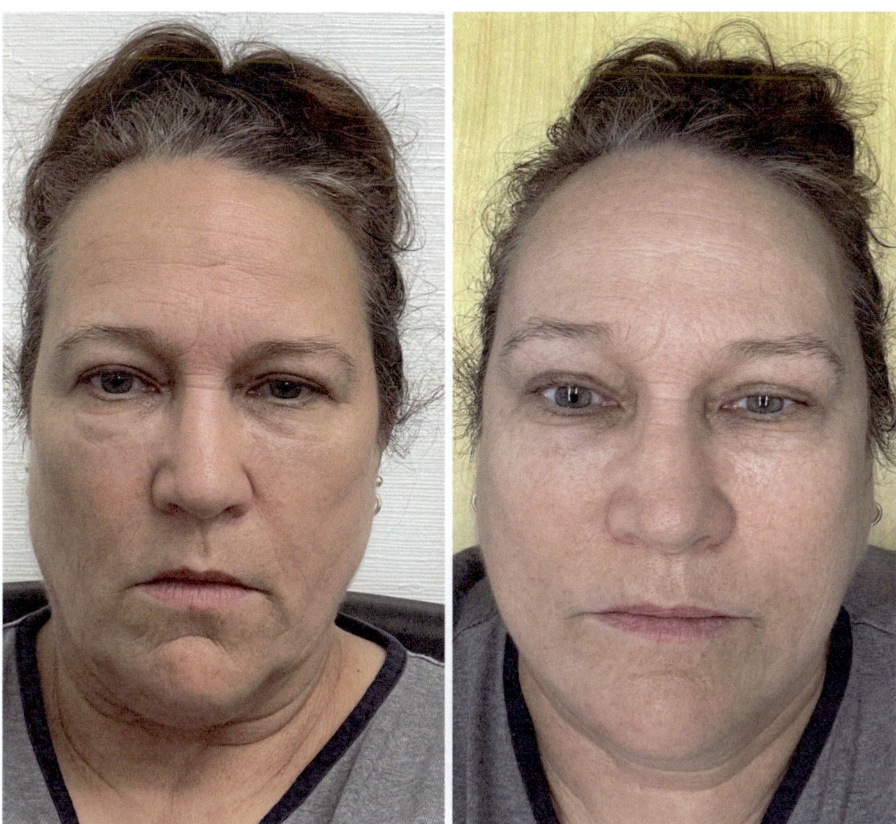

Fig. 5.2 Image of face showing improvement of signs of aging including descended cheeks and jowls when supine (on right) compared to upright (left)

centrally and inferiorly with the tissues of the periphery. Approximation of the displaced tissue closes the gaps, supports the stretched ligaments and skin, and provides a type of "internal splint" or in the case of threads more accurately "suture" to hold tissues in place while collagenesis and remodeling takes place during the subsequent months. How the barbed sutures approximate tissues that has been separated by loss of collagen and volume can be demonstrated on a pig skin model which most closely resembles human skin. Figure 5.3 shows two intact pig skin models that are marked to show that initially the markings are at equal distances from each other. When the pig skin model that is already more plump and appears to have healthier skin has its skin undermined with removal of some tissue, it can be shown that the skin overall becomes thinner and flatter (Fig. 5.4). In addition, the distance between the markings has also now increased in comparison to the intact pig skin model (Fig. 5.5). This is like what happens as aging occurs in human skin. The skin spreads, descends, prolapses, and thins. In fact, analogous to how the

Fig. 5.3 Intact pig skin
models with markings at
equal distances from each
other

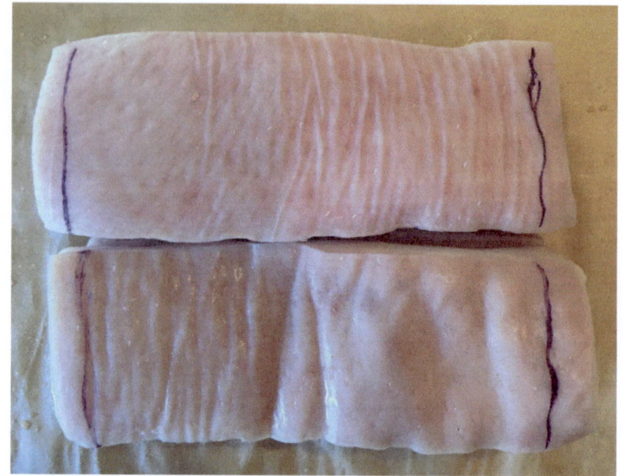

Fig. 5.4 Pig skin model
with undermined tissue is
now thinner, flatter, with
distance between markings
now greater than the intact
pig skin located behind it

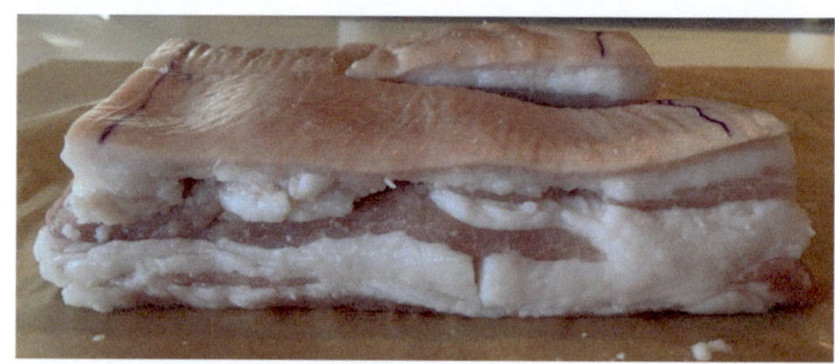

Fig. 5.5 Distance between
markers is now longer in
the pig skin model of aged
skin (lower) versus intact
pig skin (upper)

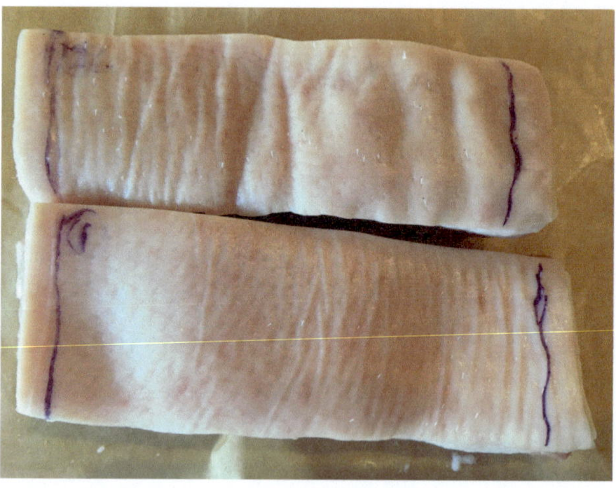

Fig. 5.6 Pig skin model with undermined tissue shown with thread placed but not yet pulled tight to approximate the tissues and close the gaps

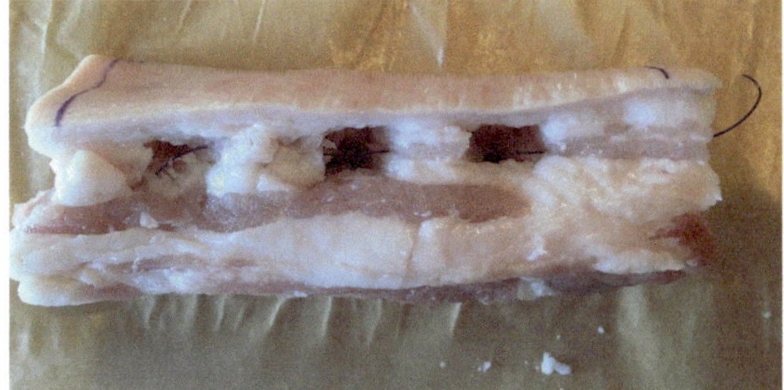

Fig. 5.7 Distance between the markings on the pig skin model with tissue approximation from threads is again now near equal to distance of the markings on the intact pig skin model

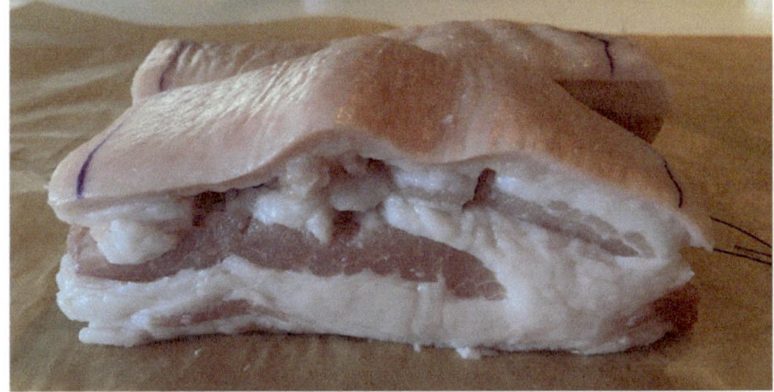

distance between the markings increase in the pig skin model, birthmarks on human skin have been shown to change their relative position on the face with aging. While in the pig skin model, the gaps are completely empty for demonstration purposes, in the human live skin, the gap may not be completely empty but is deficient and has remaining overlying skin that is stretched over the gap. In Fig. 5.6, the pig skin model for aging is shown with a thread inserted under the skin but not yet pulled tight to approximate the tissues closer together. Figure 5.7 shows on this same pig skin model that when the threads are pulled to approximate the tissue closer to one another, the gaps are closed and the skin becomes thicker and more plump again. The distance between the markings on the pig skin model for aging after the threads are pulled is now near equal to the intact pig skin model seen above it in Fig. 5.8. The threads are used to approximate the edges of the gaps, providing the "splint" needed to allow closure and remodeling of the gap. For human skin as well, the threads thus can be used to provide the approximation of tissue needed to allow remodeling, contraction of skin, and repositioning of centrally and inferiorly prolapsed tissues closer to the tissues of the periphery of the face.

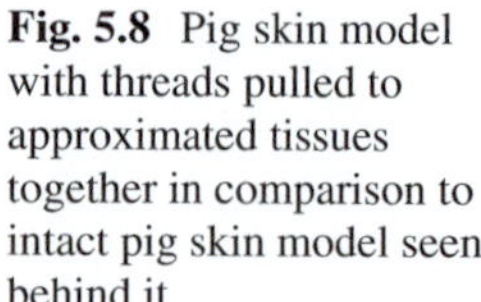

Fig. 5.8 Pig skin model with threads pulled to approximated tissues together in comparison to intact pig skin model seen behind it

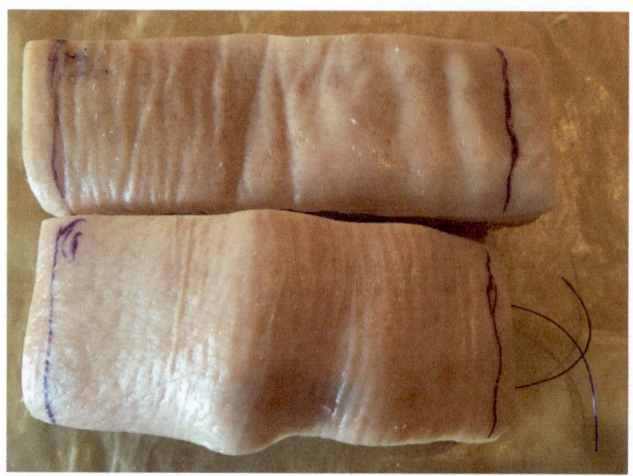

Reference

Wulc AE, et al. Anatomic basis of mid-facial aging. In: Hartstein M, et al., editors. Midfacial rejuvenation. New York, NY: Springer; 2012. p. 15–28.

Chapter 6
Variations of Threads

There are many different types of threads with different sizes and modifications. They are used for different purposes and different areas of the body (See Table 6.1). In addition, different threads may be more suitable for different face and skin types (See Table 6.2). The kinds of threads available differ by manufacturer although there are similarities between them. Since specific details and names will vary between different companies as well as between different countries, this section will not be an exhaustive account of all the different types available but will be a general overview. The threads discussed will be mono threads, spiral threads, mesh threads, barbed threads, and nose threads. There will also be information about threads of different molecular composition including Polydioxanone (PDO), Polycaprolactone (PCL), and Poly-L-Lactic Acid (PLLA).

6.1 Mono Threads

These are very thin threads generally ranging from 23 to 30 gauge. They are characterized by being smooth and flat rather than barbed or twisted (Fig. 6.1). The length can vary from very short 15 mm to as long as 60 mm. Most commonly they are loaded on sharp needles in order to ease insertion since usually a large number of them are placed in one area. Some are loaded on a cannula in order to ease placement over bony structures or to decrease risk of bruising in thin skin areas such as near the eye. These are placed generally in the upper subcutaneous layer. They are smooth on the surface having no barbs and no alteration in texture and lie completely flat once inserted. They are useful simply to stimulate collagen thereby improving the skin texture. They do not perform any movement of tissue. They are perhaps the easiest to insert as it is just a matter of simply sliding the needle or cannula under the skin and once the needle or cannula is removed the thread remains in place. There is virtually no risk of dumpling. There is, however, more risk of

© The Author(s), under exclusive license to Springer Nature
Switzerland AG 2023
N. M. Kim, *Non-Surgical Thread Procedures*,
https://doi.org/10.1007/978-3-031-36468-6_6

Table 6.1 Types of threads and their Functions

Type of thread	Common uses and function
Mono thread	For mild collagen stimulation, skin brightening, mild-moderate skin tightening, mild-moderate fat reduction, and cellulite improvement. Multiple sessions needed for more significant improvement in skin thickness may be required. Does not provide any significant repositioning of soft tissue. Can be used in all areas of face and body.
Spiral Thread	For more collagen stimulation than mono threads and mild volumization. Does not provide direct repositioning of soft tissue. Ideal for necklace lines and lip vermillion border. May be used in all areas of the face and body.
Mesh Thread	For significant collagen stimulation and volumization that is comparable to filler efficacy. Can be used in areas where building of volume and definition is desired. Ideal for brow bone, temples, undereye tear troughs, cheeks, nasolabial folds, marionette lines, chin, skin tightening for crepey skin. May be preferable for very thin patients instead of barbed threads.
Barbed/ Cog/ Molded Thread	For repositioning of soft tissue on face and body as well as significant collagen stimulation. Ideal for eyebrows lifting, cheeks and jowls repositioning, and submental neck laxity improvement.
HIKO or Nose Threads	Specialized threads for nose elevation and definition, only to be used for nose procedures.

Table 6.2 Thread recommendations for different patient face and skin types

Face and skin type	Recommended threads to consider
Thin skin with very little fatty tissue, hollowing more than sagging skin, patient with thin body habitus.	Recommend mesh threads first to thicken skin. These patients may not need barbed thread for cheeks and jowls at all but if still desired or needed the barbed threads will perform better after skin is thickened from the mesh threads. 21 gauge barbed threads if barbed threads desired.
Thick skin, heavy laxity with fat descent or accumulation.	18 gauge barbed threads to lift and reposition tissue at deeper layer. In addition, 21 gauge barbed threads inserted in more superficial fat layer to promote shrinkage of fat layer.
Average thickness skin and moderate laxity.	21 or 19 gauge barbed threads to lift and reposition tissue. 21 gauge if thinner skin and more fat loss.
Early skin aging, mainly for prevention or if collagen desired	Monothreads or spiral threads. Mesh threads as well in localized areas where early signs of aging such as thinning undereye skin.

bruising with the threads that are loaded on sharp needles. These threads are ideal for areas of skin where barbed threads would not be appropriate. They are versatile in that they can be placed in nearly any area of the skin. However, caution must be taken in terms of setting expectations for patients. These will not provide the dramatic changes in face shape or sagging. These threads require multiple applications over several months period in order to optimize improvement in the quality of the skin. It is best to do sessions 1 month apart for at least three sessions or more. It is

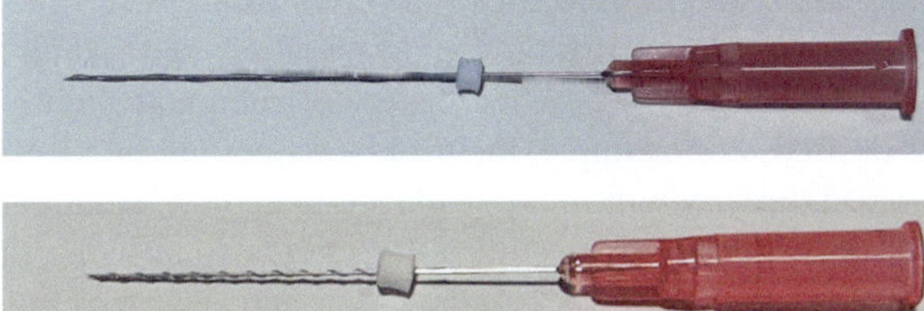

Fig. 6.1 Mono thread loaded on needle

Fig. 6.2 Spiral or twist thread loaded on needle

best to use as many threads as possible. They can be placed in a cross hatch pattern to increase the number of threads and provide more coverage. It is recommended that the threads are inserted as close as possible next to each other in order to induce collagen in the skin uniformly. The threads will serve as a scaffold for growth of collagen so more threads will maximize the degree of collagen stimulation.

The mono threads are an alternative for patients who are fearful of having barbed or cog threads placed, however, patient selection and expectation must be handled carefully. For example, anyone with even mildly sagging jowls and expects the jowls to be improved will be disappointed. Instead, mono threads would be best for patients who have very thin skin and no jowls but would like improvement in their skin quality. They would be useful also in patients who have very little fat and such thin skin such that cogged threads may not hold in their skin. The mono threads can be used in these patients to prepare the skin so that it is thicker and may hold barbed or cogged threads better.

These threads are indeed also more versatile because they can be placed on a cannula. When they are on a loaded on a cannula, a small pilot hole must be made with a needle in order to be able to pass the cannula into the skin. Since these are not loaded on a sharp needle, they can be used in areas that are bony such as for skin over knees, elbows, hands. They can also be used around the eyes such as the upper or lower lid where using needles would be more dangerous and lead to bruising.

6.2 Spiral or Twist Threads

These are like the mono threads, however, instead of lying flat they are usually in a curled shape (Fig. 6.2). They are loaded on a needle and can be seen wrapping around the needle in a tighter curl or spiral pattern such that when the thread is unloaded from the needle it will lay in the skin in a spiral pattern rather than lying flat. This shape allows for placement of more thread material and occupies more space within the skin. Thus, there is a bit more stimulation of collagen and filling than the mono threads. They generally are available in different lengths ranging from 38 to 90 mm and in different thicknesses ranging from 25 to 29 gauge. They are similarly as easy to insert as the mono threads and have very low risk of dumpling or irregularity. They are inserted in the same upper subcutaneous layer. Since they are loaded on needles, they also may cause bruising. Downtime otherwise is minimal with usually only mild swelling and redness lasting 1–2 days. They are suitable for areas where increased collagen and slightly more volume in a focal area is desired. For example, the necklace lines are an ideal location. The threads will be placed directly within the necklace lines in a linear pattern. The spiral threads help fill the depth of the necklace lines faster than mono threads. They are also helpful for patients who are extremely thin and desire to build a mild amount of overall volume in their skin over their entire face. The amount of volume developed would not approach that of filler, however, so managing patients' expectations is important when discussing this as an option. If a greater amount of volume is needed, then the mesh or braided threads would be an alternative to filler. The spiral threads can also be helpful to use in patients who are either wary of the cogged or barbed threads or would not yet be able to have success with cogged threads due to the thin nature of their skin.

6.3   Mesh Threads

These are sometimes referred to also as volumizing, braided or Boost threads. They are different names for a category of similar threads where several mono threads are braided together to form a shape that is like a thick rope (see Fig. 6.3). These allow for significantly more collagen production than the mono or the spiral threads. The amount of volume enhancement due to collagen production achieved can be comparable to filler. Thus, these threads are ideal to use in locations such as the nasolabial folds, the tear trough, the upper cheek, the marionette lines, and chin. They can also be used in the temple areas, the brow bone as well as the jawline. In contrast to the mono or spiral threads, the mesh threads have very low risk of bruising as they are always loaded on a cannula. They are thick being usually 19 gauge and can vary in length from 38 to 60 mm in length. Unlike, mono threads and spiral threads the mesh or braided threads, do not need to have repeated application to have optimal results. One treatment every 12 months should suffice for most patients. Initial changes are noticeable in the immediate period; however, the final result is most dramatically noticeable 2 months after the procedure at which time the collagen has been built up significantly. The results can be quite rewarding. The volumizing effect is indeed comparable to dermal filler but with advantages. The mesh or braided threads create skin tightening as well as volumization so avoids the excessive plumping effect of dermal fillers that is seen in some cases. These are ideal in patients who have lax thin skin that may otherwise require large amounts of dermal filler to see significant improvement. Since the threads stimulate collagen naturally

Fig. 6.3 Mesh or braided
or volume thread

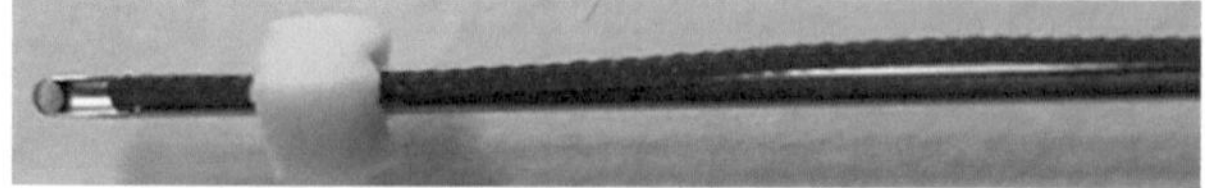

there is also less risk of undesirable shaping, placement, or contour irregularity as can occur due to side effects of injection with dermal fillers. For example, in the undereye tear trough area, with dermal fillers there is a high incidence of swelling or excessive irregularity due to filler migration. However, with the mesh or braided threads there is no filling substance other than the patient's natural collagen that is produced due to stimulation by the threads. And if the threads are placed correctly the threads are not visible under the skin. These are also ideal for patients who are fearful of the recovery period after barbed or cog threads since there is only minimal discomfort after the threads are inserted. These threads cause very little downtime since there is only a small hole made from the puncture site which heals within 1 week. There is no required limitation of oral movements with insertion of these threads during the immediate recovery period as there is with the barbed or cogged threads. In the author's personal experience the satisfaction level of these threads is very high among patients. These threads allow for more expanded versatility compared to dermal filler. For example, creation of brow bone definition which is difficult to esthetically create with dermal filler by hand is naturally produced by the mesh threads. They can in some cases be used in place of barbed or cog threads. In those cases, they would provide the advantages of no risk of dimpling and much less downtime.

6.4   Barbed or Cog Threads

Barbed or Cog threads have a surface that is not smooth but either have cuts to create a barbed surface or molded to have cog shapes on the surface. These modifications create the ability to be held strongly within soft tissue such that when the external end is pulled, it will not easily release. The barbs or cogs can be positioned bidirectional, in different directions on one end versus the other, or unidirectional. Because of the barbs or cogs' ability to affix itself into the soft tissue, it is possible to have an anchoring end and a pulling end (see Figs. 6.4 and 6.5). These are the threads traditionally thought of as creating the thread "lift." These threads can mechanically reposition skin relative to the underlying muscle layer. Therefore depending on which direction the threads are placed and approximating the skin at the pulling end towards the skin at the anchoring end, redistributing heavier tissue to create a more uniform contour is possible. It important to keep this in mind when performing the procedure. Approximation by pulling the skin together so that the skin at the pulling end is closer to the skin at the anchoring end must be performed. Even though skin may appear more dimpled, bunched or folded after the approximation, these will be usually temporary side effects if moderate. It is not as effective to simply insert the threads without performing the

Fig. 6.4 Cog thread
magnified

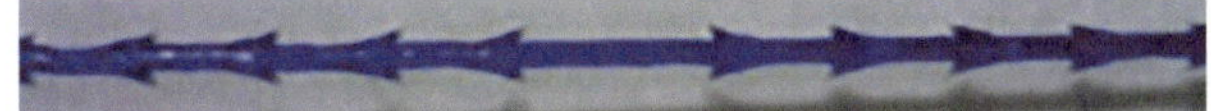

Fig. 6.5 Barbed thread magnified

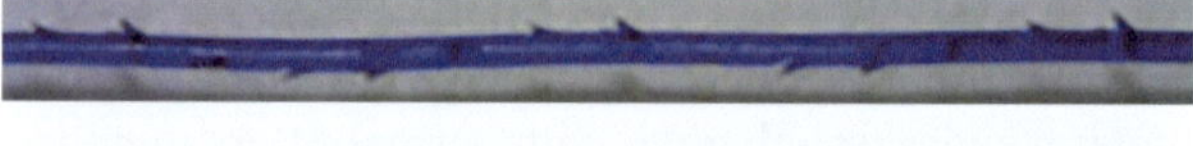

Fig. 6.6 Resculpt medical threads' three different types of cannulas with their threads loaded: Types W, D and L

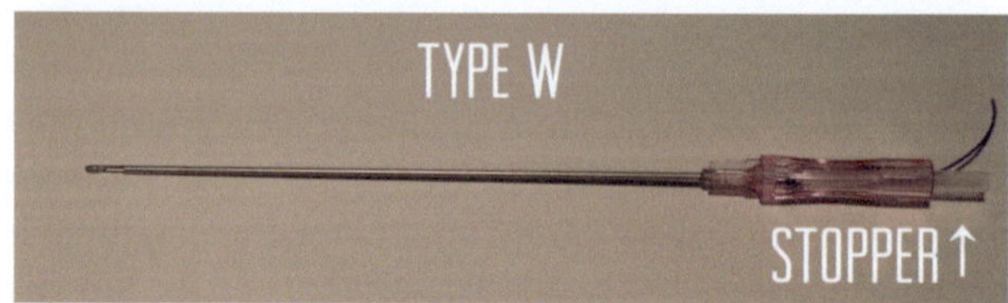

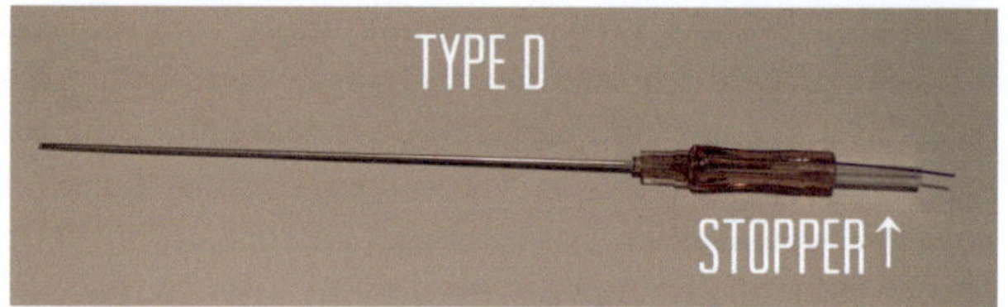

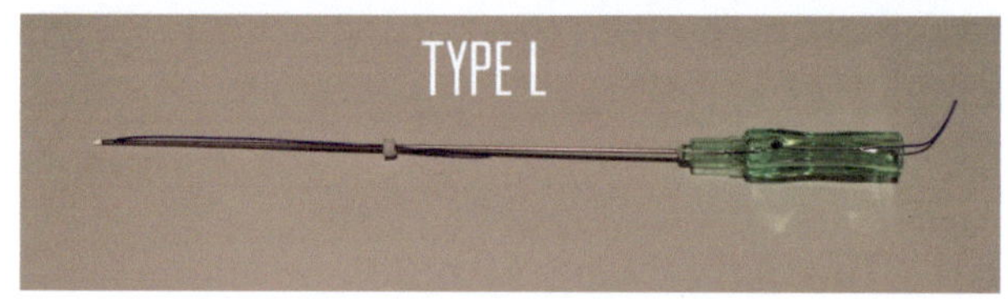

approximation of skin even though insertion alone will initially cause the skin to appear smooth and tighter due to temporary swelling. If only insertion is done, after the swelling and recovery period is over, the face, for example, will return to its original sagging shape and the patient will be disappointed. The maneuvers to approximate the skin is best learned with hands-on training and experience to feel comfortable and confident.

These threads are optimal for repositioning of the cheeks and jowls. They are also useful for repositioning of the forehead skin so that the eyebrows and eyelids are in closer approximation relative to the hairline. These threads can also be used in some body areas to help reposition flesh, however, results may significantly vary between individuals as body habitus can have a very wide spectrum of body weight whereas the spectrum is narrower in the facial area.

These threads come in different sizes usually ranging from 18 to 23 gauge. The lengths can vary as well ranging usually from 60 to 100 mm. They are loaded inside cannulas that can have varying tips. The main three types of tips available from the brand Resculpt Medical Threads, for example, are type W, type D, and type L (see Figs. 6.6 and 6.7). Type W is a smooth tip cannula with the thread end completely inside the cannula. This allows for insertion of the cannula as well as retraction since there is no external thread to snag on tissue. This is a safer cannula to use when inserting thicker gauge threads such as 18 gauge since it allows one to reposition if the first pass is not at the correct level. Also, since it has a blunt end, there is

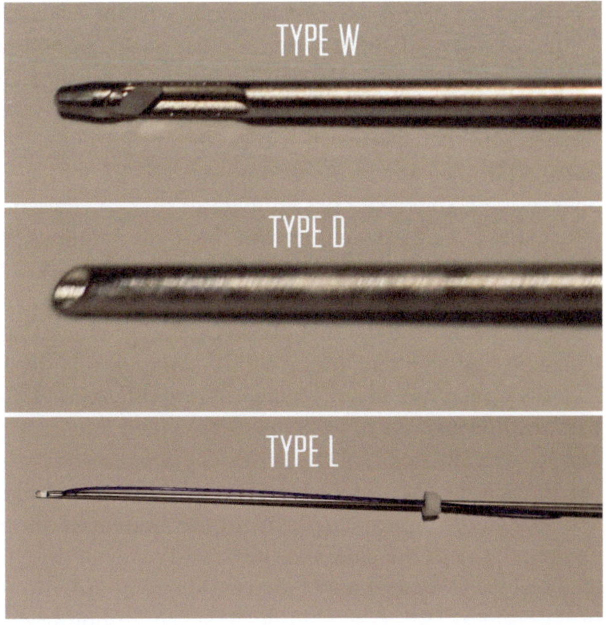

Fig. 6.7 Magnification of the tips of the three different types of cannulas loaded with threads: Types W, D and L

less risk of puncturing vessels which is important for thicker cannulas. Type D cannula also has the thread completely within the cannula and therefore also allows for repositioning of the cannula if initially inserted incorrectly. In addition, type D has a sharper end that is useful if need to insert through scar tissue or need more precise targeting of fatty pouches. It is primarily for use with thinner thread gauge such as 20 gauge or thinner. Notice that both type W and type D have a stopper at the hub that holds the thread in place (see Fig. 6.6). This stopper is removed once the cannula is in the proper location in the skin. Then the thread is pushed out through the tip so that it can attach to the tissue by tapping on the thread end at the hub. Both type W and type D are useful and may be preferred for those practitioners who are less experienced and need a more forgiving cannula that allows retraction if need to reposition the thread into the correct location or level. Notice type L, however, has some portion of thread located outside of the tip (see Figs. 6.6 and 6.7). This portion of thread is barbed or cogged so once it is inserted into the skin, it will attach to tissue and thus will remain in place even if the cannula is retracted. Thus, only a single attempt for correct placement of the thread is possible. This type is best for thinner threads such as 21 or 23 gauge since they are easier to loosen and any dimpling resolves more readily even when placed incorrectly. The tip is also blunt which allows for less risk of bruising. These, however, may be less suitable for new practitioners who are learning to correctly insert threads since they allow for only a single try. If the placement is incorrect with the initial insertion, indeed, the thread now fixated into the skin will need to be pulled out which can cause some discomfort to the patient and waste of thread.

The gauge of the thread determines what layer would be optimal for placement. The thicker threads with lower number gauge should be placed deeper within subcutaneous tissue whereas the thinner higher gauge threads can be placed more superficially within subcutaneous tissue for optimal performance. Different gauge threads will be appropriate for different patients of different skin quality (see Table 6.2). The lower gauge thicker threads will be preferred for patients with heavier jowls or heavier tissues and thicker skin. Patients with thinner skin and more laxity would be better suited with the higher number gauge or thinner threads such as the 21 or 23 gauge. Decision about which thickness of thread to use can also depend on which part of the face the threads are placed. For example, the thicker stronger threads are optimal to use for the submental laxity in the neck. The neck is a challenging area and, in the author's experience, can tolerate thicker threads such as the 18 gauge to ensure strong hold and maximize increase in collagen. Thicker threads, however, need to be used by skilled hands. A feel for when you are in the correct area and depth of tissue must be developed. The ability to drape the skin over the threads evenly should be developed to reduce significant dumpling or thread appearance. It is normal to have a small amount of dimpling or bunching depending on the quality of the patient's skin. Mild cases of dimpling and bunching will spontaneously resolve and may be unavoidable in order to ensure optimal repositioning of the tissues. However, significant severe dimpling due to poor thread placement, particularly too superficial placement, will be painful for the patient and may take many months for resolution or may not completely resolve.

6.5 Nose Threads

Threads used in the nose are specially designed only for use in the nose. There are two kinds. One is shorter generally 19 gauge with a length of 38 mm. The 38 mm length is folded in half so that it is strong and will fit in the columella of the nose (see Fig. 6.8). These act as a kind of "strut" to lift the nose tip. The other kind is designed to build height to the bridge of the nose. These are generally 19 gauge and of the length of 50 mm (see Fig. 6.9). The lengths and configuration of loading on the cannulas of both types of nose threads are such that the entire length of the thread will be inserted when the cannula is completely inserted. There should be no end of thread remaining outside of the insertion hole. They both have barbs or cogs to help the thread stay inside the skin when the cannulas are retracted (See Fig. 6.10).

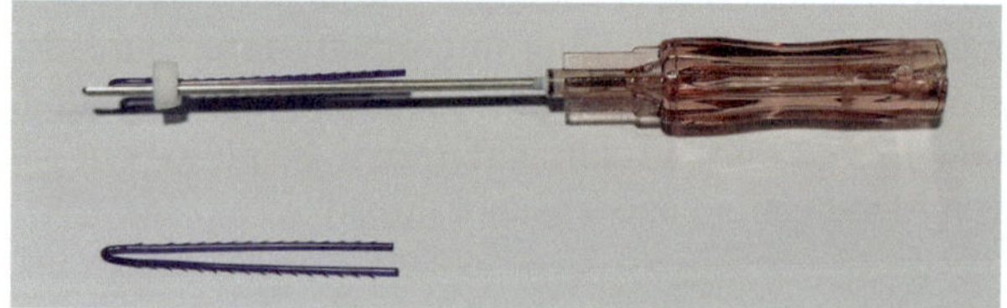

Fig. 6.8 19 gauge × 38 mm Nose thread for columella shown loaded on the cannula (upper) and outside of the cannula (lower)

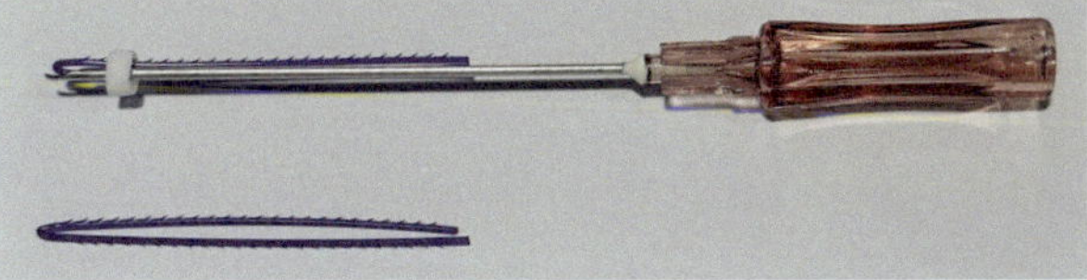

Fig. 6.9 19 gauge × 50 mm Nose thread for bridge shown loaded on the cannula (upper) and outside the cannula (lower)

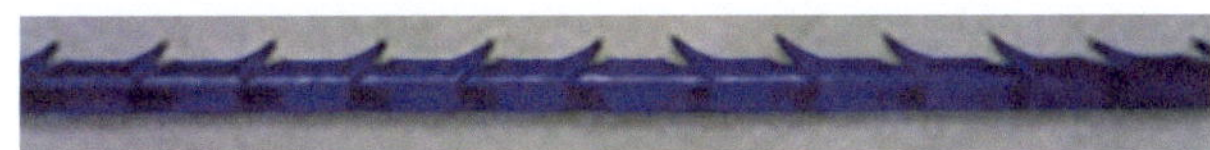

Fig. 6.10 Barbs on nose threads magnified

Table 6.3 Different types of thread composition

	PDO	PCL	PLLA	PCL/PLLA
Duration until absorption	6–8 months	12–18 months	12 months	14–18 months
Stiffness and Foreign Body Sensation	Moderate	Low	High	Moderate
Flexibility	Moderate	High	Low	Moderate
Advantages	Comfortable Whitening/ Brightening effect	Long lasting effect	Long lasting effect and strength of threads	Long lasting effect with comfort and less risk of breakage
Disadvantages	Not as long duration of effect although with collagen stimulation effective duration can be 1 year	Higher risk of breakage due to softness/ flexibility. Not yet FDA Approved for soft tissue approximation	Can feel stiff for patient.	Not yet FDA approved for soft tissue approximation.

6.6   Different Compositions of Threads

Although in the USA, polydioxanone (PDO) is the chemical composition of the threads that are primarily used and have gained FDA recognition for cosmetic purposes, in other countries threads of other composition are gaining in popularity. In particular, a thread that is a copolymer of two different components have combined the best traits of both to provide optimal performance. This thread is composed of both Polycaprolactone and Poly-L-lactic acid. It may have a different abbreviation depending on the manufacturer, but PCL-PLLA or PLCL are commonly used. While the Poly-L-lactic acid component provides a longer lasting effect, the Polycaprolactone mitigates the stiffness of pure Poly-L-lactic acid to offer a more comfortable feeling in the skin (see Table 6.3). The PCL-PLLA threads can have a duration of 18 months while still be tolerated well by the patient. For the remainder of this textbook, unless otherwise stated, threads referred to will be specifically PDO or polydioxanone threads since those are FDA approved in the USA.

Chapter 7
Insertion Technique for Barbed or Cog Threads

7.1 Supplies

(a) Alcohol or other anti-septic cleanser
(b) 18-gauge needle
(c) 30-gauge needle
(d) 100-mm 22-gauge cannula (for face and neck) or 60 mm 25-gauge cannula (for eyebrows)
(e) 22-gauge needle or other size to draw up anesthetic
(f) 1.0 cc syringe
(g) 2% lidocaine with epinephrine
(h) 8.4% Sodium Bicarbonate for injection
(i) Iris scissors and forceps (or suture removal kit)
(j) Alcohol gel
(k) White cosmetic pencil and flexible ruler
(l) Resculpt Medical Threads™ barbed or cog threads loaded on cannula.

7.2 Method

1. Cleanse area to be treated with makeup remover if needed and then with anti-septic cleanser.
2. Draw with the cosmetic pencil and ruler the lines for the path of insertion as desired. Subsequent chapters will cover in more detail pattern of insertion recommended for different areas.
3. Engage 22-gauge needle on syringe and draw up 0.2 cc of bicarbonate. Then fill the remainder of the 1.0 cc syringe with the 2% lidocaine with epinephrine.
4. Change the needle on the syringe to the 30-gauge needle.

© The Author(s), under exclusive license to Springer Nature Switzerland AG 2023
N. M. Kim, *Non-Surgical Thread Procedures*,
https://doi.org/10.1007/978-3-031-36468-6_7

5. Inject superficially to make a wheal of the anesthetic at one end of the line where the pilot hole for insertion of the thread will take place. The location preferred is around the periphery of the face rather than a central location. At the site of the wheal make a pilot hole with the 18 gauge needle. It is easier to puncture with the needle at a 45° or less angle rather than perpendicularly. This helps avoid puncturing any deep vessels causing more bleeding.

6. Change the needle on the syringe to the cannula.

7. Inject with the cannula on syringe the anesthetic as you advance subcutaneously through the pilot hole and along the line that was drawn.

8. Repeat this procedure for all the lines drawn in order to anesthetize all the paths along which the threads will be inserted.

9. Once anesthesia is completed thread insertion may be begun. Enter through the pilot hole and advance the thread on the cannula subcutaneously. Use the left hand to either stretch the skin as needed to have a smooth pathway of insertion as well as at times try to drape the skin over the thread. It is important to try to remain in the subcutaneous tissue or the fat layer. If you advance too superficially the thread will cause significant pain and significant dimpling.

10. Once the thread and cannula is advanced to the point desired and to the entire length of the cannula, it is time to remove the cannula. If there is a stopper in the hub of the cannula, remove it at this time then push the end of the thread through the tip until you feel that the thread barb is engaged. You can test this by pulling on the end of the thread. If the barbs are engaged then you will feel resistance to the pulling. Apply a small amount of the alcohol gel to your fingertips of the left hand. Place slight pressure with your left hand on the end tip of the cannula through the top of the skin in order to ensure engagement of the thread barbs with the tissue. As you retract the cannula slide your left hand along towards the end of the cannula in order to engage all the barbs within the tissue. The alcohol gel helps to lubricate the skin and make this a smoother maneuver. The thread should remain within the tissue automatically with this technique while the cannula is easily removed. See the Instructional Video 33.2 in Chap. 33 included with the textbook to view a demonstration.

11. Repeat this procedure with all the threads.

12. Once all the threads are inserted pull on the end of the thread that is outside of the skin while pushing the skin downwards towards the pulling end over the thread. This allows the lift of skin and approximation of the skin at the distal or pulling end towards the skin of the proximal portion or anchoring end of the thread (See Fig. 10.3 and Instructional Videos 33.2 and 33.3 in Chap. 33). This in effect causes a "lifted" appearance of sagging tissue due to approximation of the pulled end towards the anchoring end. It is important to perform this maneuver and tighten the skin even though it may cause more bunching of skin near the anchoring site. Figure 7.1 shows the difference between merely inserting the thread and not performing the approximation maneuver on one side of the face versus the other side where the approximation maneuver was performed. The maneuver may cause buckling of skin at the anchoring site but this may be necessary to have a better result of "lifting." In Fig. 10.9, the threads are merely inserted without doing the approximation maneuver, so no buckling

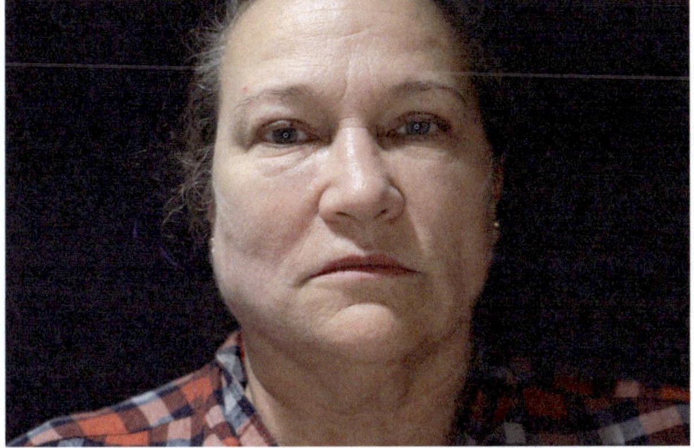

Fig. 7.1 Comparison of threads with and without approximation maneuver in procedure for cheeks and jowls treatment. Left side of face after approximation maneuver shows more "lifted" and youthful contour while the right side of face has less change in contour after threads have been inserted but no approximation maneuver performed

is seen. While this may be more tolerable for the patient post-procedure, once the swelling and buckling resolves with recovery, the patient will likely be dissatisfied with the degree of change and feel that there was no "lift." Fig. 10.10, on the other hand, shows that after the approximation maneuver, there is buckling at the anchoring site. This buckling should be tolerated by both the practitioner and the patient as it will resolve in a few days. Because the approximation maneuver was performed, the result of a "lifted" appearance will be more pronounced.

13. Repeat this with all the threads.
14. It is helpful to raise the patient to sitting position and reevaluate the appearance and shaping or contour achieved. If there is any significant dimpling, try to remove by placing pressure through the skin at a more proximal location (see Instructional Video 33.3 in Chap. 33). Mild dimpling can be tolerated and will resolve quickly. If more lifting is desired or needed one may do this at this time as well by pulling on the end of the thread more and performing the approximation maneuver.
15. Once the desired degree of tightening and approximation of the skin has been achieved it is time to cut the end of the thread that is outside of the skin.
16. Use the forceps to hold the end of the thread while pushing down on the skin with the iris scissors to cut as closely as possible to the skin. When this is done the end of the thread should bury under the skin once the thread is cut off at the end.
17. Check with your finger to make sure that all the threads are cut short enough so that it is buried under the skin. If you feel a sharp end at the insertion site, then the thread was not cut short enough. Use the forceps again to try to pull the end of the thread and cut again as closely as possible while pushing down on the skin to cut deeply. Alternatively, you may try to push the skin over the end of the thread so that the thread becomes buried.
18. Apply antibiotic ointment on the insertion sites.
19. Prescribe prophylactic antibiotics such as Minocycline 100 mg twice a day for 7 days.

Chapter 8
Insertion Technique for Mesh Threads

8.1 Supplies

(a) Alcohol or other anti-septic cleanser.
(b) 2% Lidocaine with Epinephrine
(c) 8.4% Sodium Bicarbonate for injection
(d) 18-gauge needle
(e) 22-gauge needle
(f) 23, 25, or 27-gauge cannula 60-mm length
(g) 30-gauge needle
(h) 1.0 cc syringe
(i) Gauze
(j) White cosmetic pencil for drawing
(k) Flexible ruler
(l) Resculpt Medical Threads™ 19-gauge by 38-mm or 60-mm length mesh Boost thread.

8.2 Method

1. Remove all makeup and cleanse the area with alcohol or other antiseptic cleanser.
2. Use ruler and white cosmetic pencil to draw the lines with proper length along the paths that thread is planned to be inserted. This will be dependent on the area that needs to be addressed and corrected. Subsequent chapters will cover the pattern of insertions that is recommended for the different areas.

© The Author(s), under exclusive license to Springer Nature Switzerland AG 2023

N. M. Kim, *Non-Surgical Thread Procedures*,
https://doi.org/10.1007/978-3-031-36468-6_8

3. Engage the 22-gauge needle on the 1.0 cc syringe. Use this to draw up 0.2 cc of the bicarbonate and 0.8 cc of the 2% lidocaine with epinephrine in the same syringe.

4. Change the needle on the syringe to the 30-gauge needle.

5. At the end of the drawn lines where insertion of the thread is planned make a small superficial wheal with the anesthetic using the 30-gauge needle and syringe.

6. Change the needle on the syringe to the cannula.

7. With the 18-gauge needle make a puncture at the site of the wheal of anesthetic. In order to avoid inadvertent puncture of deeper lying vessels angle the needle 45° or less rather than inserting perpendicularly.

8. Enter this puncture site with the cannula attached to the syringe and as you advance inject small amounts of anesthetic along the line that was drawn thereby anesthetizing the path that the thread will be inserted along.

9. Repeat this procedure for all areas that insertion of the thread is planned.

10. Once all the areas are anesthetized, insertion of the actual threads may be begun.

11. Insert the mesh thread by entering through the entry hole. It is helpful to rotate or twist the cannula on which the thread is loaded in order to ease overcoming resistance of the tissues. Do not push too hard but instead try to drape the skin over the thread at the same time to aid advancement of the cannula. Be sure to advance to the entire length of the cannula and then slightly further to ensure that the thread will be completely under the skin (see Instructional Video 33.2 in Chap. 33).

12. In order to remove the cannula and ensure that the thread stays within the tissues, place some pressure on the skin that now has the cannula and thread within it with your left hand where the tip would be. In some cases, this is extremely important as when the skin is lax the thread may not stay completely within the tissue and a small portion of the end will remain outside of the entry hole. If this happens the thread must be completely removed, and the insertion attempted again with a new cannula and thread. In patients who have tight skin this is usually not an issue.

13. Repeat this insertion of threads at all the sites that have been anaesthetized.

14. Apply antibiotic ointment to all entry sites to promote faster healing.

Chapter 9
Insertion Technique for Mono Threads

9.1 Supplies

(a) Alcohol or other anti-septic cleanser
(b) 2% Lidocaine with Epinephrine
(c) 8.4% Sodium Bicarbonate for injection
(d) 18-gauge needle
(e) 22-gauge needle
(f) 23, 25, or 27-gauge cannula of length appropriate for size of area to be treated
(g) 30-gauge needle
(h) 1.0 cc syringe
(i) Gauze
(j) Resculpt Medical Threads™ selected for the specific area. The following chapter will describe in more detail which threads are best for which areas.

9.2 Method

1. Remove all makeup and cleanse the area with alcohol or other ant-septic cleanser.
2. Use ruler and white cosmetic pencil to outline the area that is to be treated. Subsequent chapters will cover the pattern of insertions that is recommended for the different areas.
3. Engage the 22-gauge needle on the 1.0 cc syringe. Use this to draw up 0.2 cc of the bicarbonate and 0.8 cc of the 2% lidocaine with epinephrine in the same syringe.
4. Change the needle on the syringe to the 30-gauge needle.

© The Author(s), under exclusive license to Springer Nature
Switzerland AG 2023
N. M. Kim, *Non-Surgical Thread Procedures*,
https://doi.org/10.1007/978-3-031-36468-6_9

5. In a location that will allow you to anesthetize the area outlined, make a small superficial wheal with the anesthetic using the 30-gauge needle and syringe.
6. Change the needle on the syringe to the cannula.
7. With the 18-gauge needle make a puncture at the site of the wheal of anesthetic. In order to avoid inadvertent puncture of deeper lying vessels angle the needle 45° or less rather than inserting perpendicularly.
8. Enter this puncture site with the cannula attached to the syringe and as you advance inject small amounts of anesthetic in the area that is to be treated.
9. Repeat this procedure for all areas that insertion of the thread is planned.
10. This technique is for mono threads that are loaded on needles. Therefore, there is no pilot hole needed.
11. Pattern of placement of threads may be chosen based on the location in addition to the size of the threads. A mesh pattern is ideal, if possible, to ensure uniform tightening of skin and collagen stimulation.
12. Insert the needle with loaded threads under the skin either subcutaneously or deep dermis. Insert the entire length of the needle.
13. Remove the needles after insertion. All the needles may be placed at once prior to removal, several at a time inserted and removed, or one at a time.
14. The thread should remain in the skin without any excess protruding outside of the skin. Usually with mono threads there is no need to hold down the skin to ensure that the threads stay within the tissue. If, however, the thread does not completely stay within the skin, it must be completely pulled out by the end protruding and a new insertion must be done with a new thread.
15. Avoid placing the thread too superficially otherwise slight irregularity or hyperpigmentation may result.
16. Apply pressure if any bleeding. Bruises are not uncommon with this procedure since the threads are loaded on sharp needles and the placement is relatively superficial. Particularly in areas that are highly vascular such as the neck, some bruising may be unavoidable.
17. In some areas that are rounded or curved such as the neck, the needles are thin and flexible enough that they can be manually directed to follow the curve of the skin in order to maintain the correct depth.
18. If the mono threads are loaded on cannulas rather than sharp needles, a pilot hole can be made with a needle that has a gauge that is slightly larger than the gauge of the cannulas. It is important that the pilot hole is only slightly larger otherwise the thread may extrude back out of the hole after some movement.
19. After all the threads are inserted apply antibiotic ointment to the area to promote faster healing.

Chapter 10
Procedure for Lifting Cheeks and Jowls with Barbed Threads

10.1 Cheeks

1. After cleansing draw the pattern of thread insertion depending on patients' pattern of aging.
2. Figure 10.1 shows the pattern of thread placement that is useful for most patients. This pattern helps improve the laxity in the upper anterior cheek and is appropriate also for patients who have very deep nasolabial folds.
3. In some cases, it may be better to have the second thread be even a bit more below the lip corner. This would be particularly helpful in patients who tend to have downturned mouth corners.
4. Be sure to draw the line while measuring it. It should be at least as long as the length of the cannula that you will be using while still extending to the area of lax skin that is desired to be lifted (see Instructional Video 33.1 in Chap. 33).

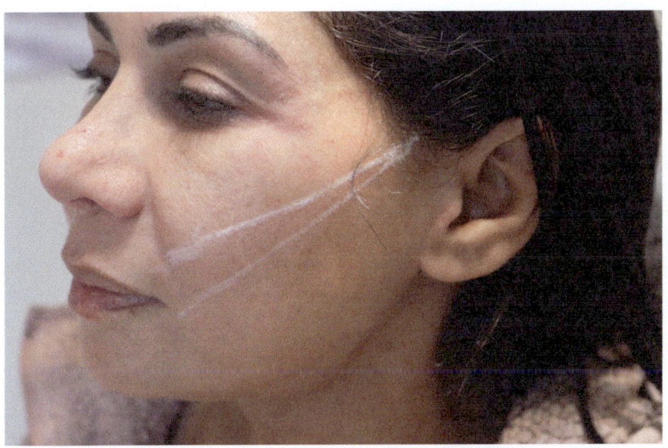

Fig. 10.1 Lines drawn for pattern of thread placement for cheeks

© The Author(s), under exclusive license to Springer Nature
Switzerland AG 2023
N. M. Kim, *Non-Surgical Thread Procedures*,
https://doi.org/10.1007/978-3-031-36468-6_10

5. Once the pattern has been drawn and decided upon, place the patient in supine position and at a level that is comfortable for the practitioner.
6. Note in Fig. 10.1 that the insertion sites should be at or near the hairline. This makes it much more comfortable for the patient in terms of downtime as the insertion hole is then easily hidden.
7. For the cheeks and jowls, the selection of thread gauge may vary depending on the skin type and thickness. For patients who have thinner, lax skin, Resculpt Medical Threads™ 21 G barbed × 90 mm may be preferable and cause less dimpling and less risk of inserting too superficially. Using a thinner thread will also ensure that you will be at the depth that will allow mobility of the skin. If using too thick thread, the barbs will hold too much to the deeper layers of skin and fascia that are less mobile. For patients who have thicker skin or more fat tissue, using 19G × 100 mm or 18G × 100 mm is recommended as the tissue will be heavier.
8. Inject the insertion site with a wheal of 2% lidocaine with epinephrine mixed with 8.4% Sodium bicarbonate as described in Chap. 7 describing insertion technique for barbed threads.
9. Make a pilot entry hole with an 18-gauge needle.
10. It is preferable to start with the superior thread path and then proceed inferiorly. In other words, insert the thread along the line drawn that is higher in the face.
11. For the thread planned for insertion into the upper cheek area, because the cheekbone can make the path of insertion convex, it is helpful to put a slight curve in the cannula by bending it (See Fig. 10.2). Do this by holding the cannula with a clean gauze moistened with alcohol to enhance sterility. The curve in the cannula will make it easier to follow the curve of the cheekbone and advance the thread without advancing too superficially in the skin.
12. Curving the cannula with a bend can be utilized for the inferior thread as well if the pathway appears to have significant curvature as many faces do in the cheek area.
13. Insert all the threads without tightening or approximating tissue at first.
14. Once all the threads have been inserted, then start to gradually tighten and approximate the tissues by pulling on the end of each thread while moving the

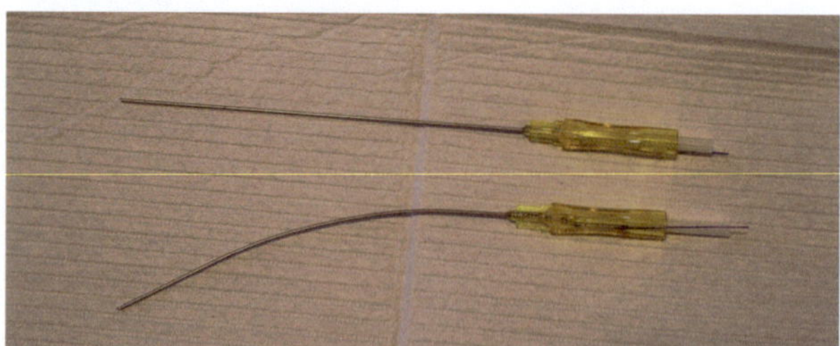

Fig. 10.2 Thread on cannula shown at top in straight original form and below bent with a slight curve to aid in placement over convex surfaces such as the cheeks

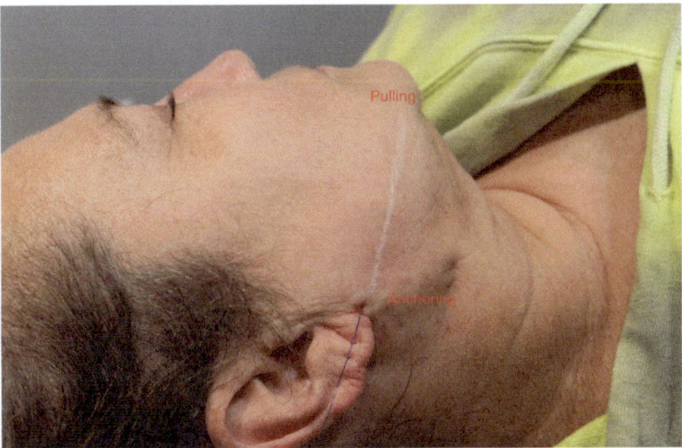

Fig. 10.3 Location of pulling end and anchoring end of thread after insertion

tissue at the anchoring end down towards the tissue at the pulling end (See Fig. 10.3). See Instructional Videos 33.2 and 33.3 in Chap. 33 for a demonstration of the procedure.

15. Avoid tightening and lifting too much to avoid excessive dimpling and buckling. However, tighten and pull enough to get an improvement in the contour of the face that is appealing and as symmetrical as possible.

16. Then raise the patient to a sitting position. Reassess the face contours and the skin for excessive dimpling. Tighten and lift more if needed for symmetry or for more improvement of laxity.

17. If there is excessive dimpling, attempt to remove it by placing some pressure more proximal to the anchoring end to try to release some of the skin from the barbs (see Instructional Video 33.3 in Chap. 33). This technique will be described further in a subsequent chapter. For this technique it is also necessary to watch a demonstration in order to fully understand the technique. And of course, hands on experience is paramount.

18. Once the positioning of the threads and tightness is satisfactory, cut the ends of the threads at the anchoring end one at a time. Ensure that you push down on the skin as much as possible while cutting in order to avoid leaving excess thread outside of the skin. If the thread is cut closely enough down on the skin, the end of the thread will bury itself under the skin. If it does not bury, apply some pressure to release some of the skin from the barbs so that it can cover the end of the thread. It is possible to check that the thread is not sticking out of the skin by placing your finger on the hole and feeling for any sharpness.

19. Place antibiotic ointment on the insertion sites. Gently wipe away any remaining pencil marks with alcohol.

20. Prescribe prophylactic antibiotics such as minocycline 100 mg bid for 7 days.

21. Advise the patient that final results are seen in 2 months after the procedure. Significant change in skin quality including thickening and increase in tautness

occur due to the collagen stimulation. This process allows for a more lifted appearance. Figure 10.11 shows an example of the before and after change in contour of cheeks and jowls one month after thread lift with barbed threads.

10.2   Jowls

1. After cleansing draw the pattern of thread insertion depending on patient's current state of aging.
2. Figure 10.4 shows the recommended pattern of thread placement for treatment of jowls. Generally, three threads on each side is optimal. However, in some patients with mild laxity only two threads may be sufficient. Patients with more laxity may require more threads. Results for the jowl are optimal if cheeks are also treated at the same time. Figure 10.5 illustrates a pattern for both combined. Also see Instructional Video 33.1 in Chap. 33 for a demonstration of the pattern of thread placement determination.
3. It is important for the most inferiorly located thread to be along the inferior part of the mandible itself. This thread should not be omitted as it gives much better results.
4. It is important to have a separate insertion hole for each thread, particularly the inferior thread. Otherwise, there is too much swelling over the angle of the jaw creating a very square appearance in the immediate post-procedure period. Although this swelling does resolve after 1–2 weeks, patients tend to be anxious about and dislike this appearance. When each thread has its own insertion hole all the tissue is pulled across evenly rather than gathered between two threads from a single insertion hole.
5. When drawing the pattern of the threads it is important to not draw past the marionette line. If the thread is placed too far past the marionette line it could make the jowls bunch up more rather than pulling the jowls posteriorly.

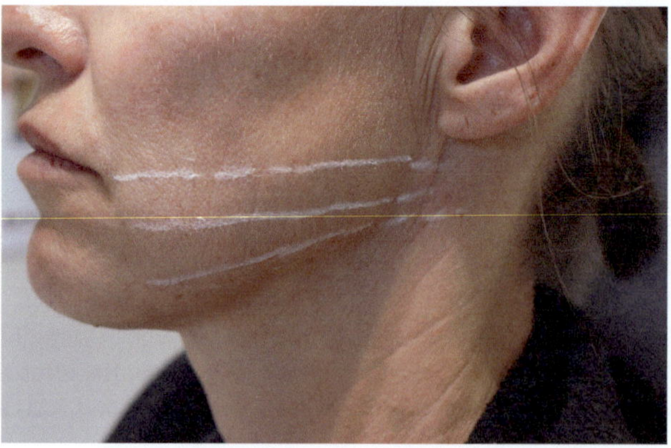

Fig. 10.4 Lines drawn for pattern of thread placement for treatment of jowls

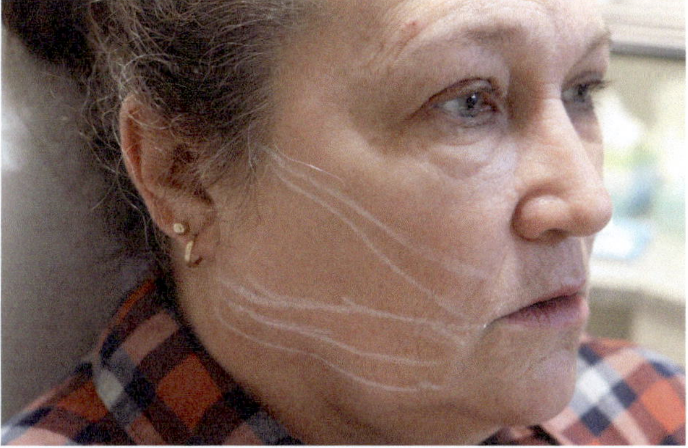

Fig. 10.5 Lines drawn for pattern of thread placement for treatment of both cheeks and jowls

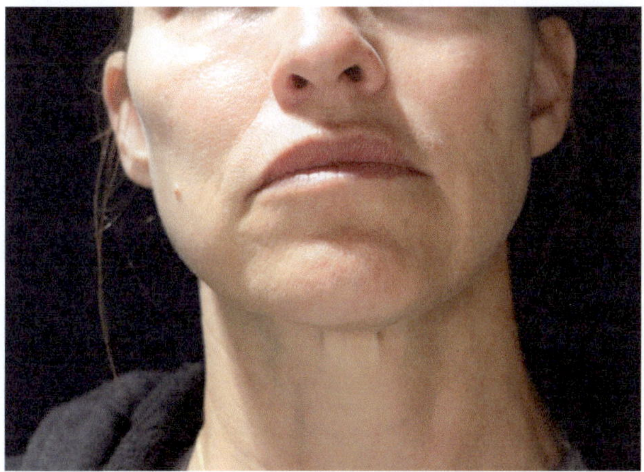

Fig. 10.6 Patient with thinner skin and face ideal for Resculpt Medical Threads™ 21 Gauge 90 mm or 100 mm barbed threads

6. Be sure to draw the line while measuring it. It should be at least as long as the length of the cannula that you will be using while still extending to the area of lax skin that is desired to be improved.

7. The size threads recommended are Resculpt Medical Threads™ 18 Gauge 100 mm barbed for thicker skin, Resculpt Medical Threads™ 19 Gauge 100mm barbed for moderate thickness skin, or 21 Gauge 90 mm barbed threads for thinner skin and smaller faces. Figure 10.6 shows a patient who would need to have 21 Gauge 100 mm threads while Figure 10.7 shows a patient who would be able to have 18 Gauge 100 mm threads with no complications.

8. Some patients benefit from two layers of thread. If patients have a significant amount of fat tissue or laxity, then a thinner thread such as 21 gauge placed more superficially in the fatty or upper subcutaneous layer can be helpful to

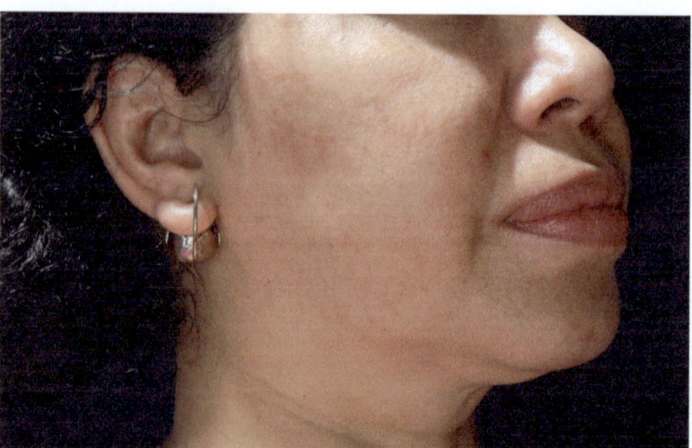

Fig. 10.7 Patient with thicker skin who can receive Resculpt Medical Threads™ 18 Gauge 100 mm barbed threads without complications

Fig. 10.8 Case where an additional layer of thinner threads for cheeks and jowls would be helpful

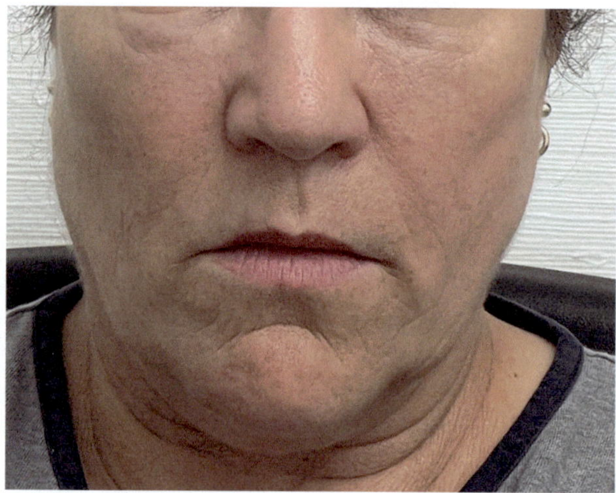

smooth the contour. In other words, 18-gauge 100-mmthreads may be used to create significant lift of the jowls. And then 21-gauge 90-mm threads can be placed more superficially in the fatty layer to promote more flattening or smoothing of skin. Figure 10.8 shows a case where adding an additional layer of thinner threads would be helpful. Note that with thinner threads, the length is usually shorter as in this case. The 21-gauge thread cannulas may be only 90 mm long. Therefore, the insertion site would need to be on the face since not long enough to go behind the earlobe.

9. If drawn correctly the insertion holes for 100mm length threads should be behind the angle of the mandible and behind the earlobe as well. This is preferable as the holes will not be as visible compared to placing the insertion holes on the face itself. In addition, there is generally less bunching of skin that sometimes causes a swelled appearance at the angle of the mandible during the first

few days after the procedure{ }:=]. This allows for the downtime to be much more tolerable, allowing patients to return to their social routine by the next day. Patients will find it easier to hide the holes with their hair.

10. Once the pattern has been drawn and decided upon, lay the patient down so they are supine and at a level that is comfortable for the practitioner.

11. Inject the insertion sites with a wheal of 2% lidocaine with epinephrine mixed with bicarbonate as described in Chap. 7 describing insertion technique for barbed threads.

12. Make a pilot entry hole with an 18-gauge needle at the site of the wheal of anesthesia.

13. It is preferable to start with the superior thread path and then proceed inferiorly. In other words, insert the thread along the line drawn that is higher in the face.

14. Insert all the threads without tightening at first.

15. Once all the threads have been inserted, then start to gradually tighten and approximate the tissues by holding the end of the thread while pushing the tissue at the anchoring end closer to that of the pulling end. See Instructional Videos 33.2 and 33.3 in Chap. 33 for a demonstration.

16. Avoid tightening and lifting too much to avoid excessive dimpling and buckling. However, tighten enough to get an improvement in the contour of the face that is appealing and as symmetrical as possible. Do not merely insert the threads without pulling and approximating the tissue. Some dimpling and buckling is necessary to get a good result and will resolve in a few days' time. Figure 10.9 shows the skin after thread insertion, but no approximating maneuver done on thread. Figure 10.10 shows how the skin may appear after approximation demonstrating the buckling that occurs at the anchoring site that is completely appropriate and at times necessary for an adequate result. Buckling will almost always resolve in a few days, and the patient must be reassured of this.

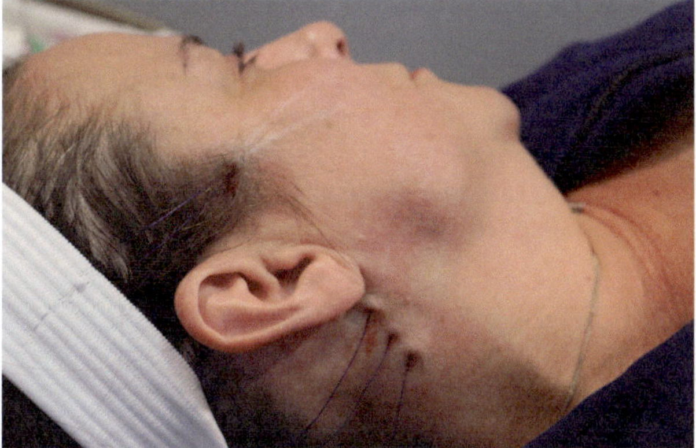

Fig. 10.9 Skin after insertion of barbed threads in jowls but before pulling approximation maneuver showing no buckling

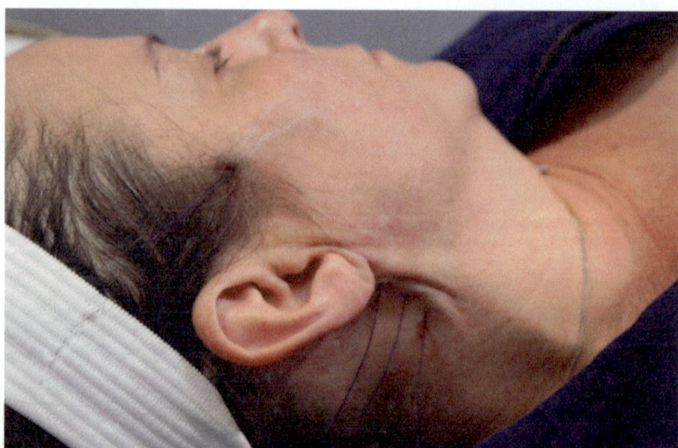

Fig. 10.10 Buckling of skin at anchoring site after insertion of barbed threads in jowls and after pulling approximation maneuver performed. This will lead to a better result than if no approximation maneuver performed

17. Once approximation has been done, raise the patient to a sitting position. Reassess the face contours and the skin for excessive dimpling. Tighten and lift more if needed for symmetry or for more improvement of laxity.
18. If there is excessive dimpling attempt to remove it by applying some pressure closer to the anchoring end of the thread to try to release some of the skin from the barbs. This technique will be described further in a subsequent chapter. It is necessary to watch a demonstration in order to fully understand the technique. And of course, hands on experience is paramount.
19. Once the positioning of the threads and tightness is satisfactory, cut the ends of the threads one at a time. Ensure that you push down on the skin as much as possible while cutting in order to avoid leaving excess thread outside of the skin. If the thread is cut closely enough down on the skin, the end of the thread will bury itself under the skin. If it does not, apply slight pressure near the hole in order to release some of the skin from the barbs so that it will cover the end of the thread. It is possible to check that the thread is not sticking out of the skin by placing your finger on the hole and feeling for any sharpness.
20. Place antibiotic ointment on the insertion sites.
21. Prescribe prophylactic antibiotics such as minocycline 100 mg bid for 7 days.
22. Figure 10.11 shows an example of change in contour of jowls one months after thread lift of cheeks and jowls with barbed threads.

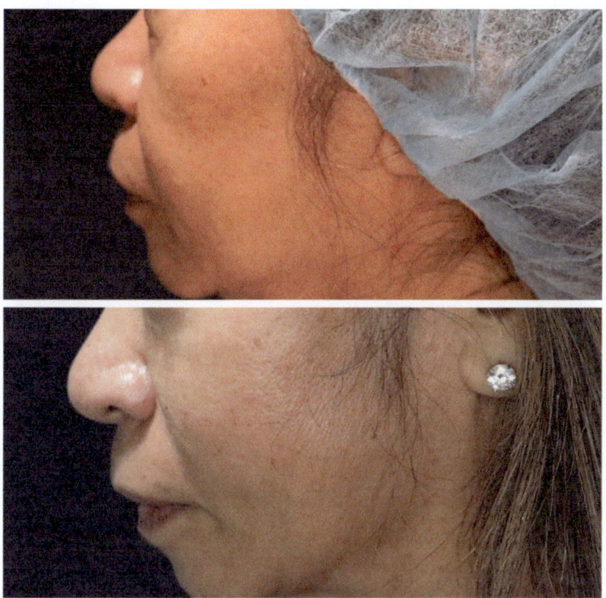

Fig. 10.11 Before and 1 month after thread lift of cheeks and jowls

Chapter 11
Procedure for Lifting Eyebrows, Eyelids, and Forehead with Barbed Threads

1. Remove makeup and cleanse the forehead with antiseptic cleanser particularly around the hairline.
2. Draw the lines with a cosmetic pencil according to the pattern of insertion desired for the threads. This requires some assessment of the patient as well as agreeing on how many threads the patient would like to have and how many would be needed for their goals.
3. The insertion site is best to be along the hairline to allow for a more comfortable down time so that the holes are not easily visible.
4. The threads that are recommended are either Resculpt Medical Threads 21 gauge or 20 gauge with a length of 60 mm with barbs or cogs.
5. Some patterns of thread placement that are useful are shown. Figure 11.1 shows a pattern that would be for a patient who primarily wants to lift the lateral eye, eyebrow, and eyelid. This is a popular procedure at this time and is referred to as the "fox eyes" on social media. Even young people have a desire for this procedure due to its popularity on social media. This pattern usually only requires 4–6 threads.
6. Figure 11.2 shows a pattern that is helpful for patients who have more laxity in the forehead and drooping of the eyelids. This pattern requires 6–8 threads.
7. Figure 11.3 shows a pattern for patients who want improvement in their lateral inferior crow's feet and sagging in this area.
8. Once the patterns are drawn lay the patient supine. When the patient is supine, forehead vessels may become engorged and more visible. Take this opportunity to trace any large vessels that are easily visible in order to help avoid puncturing any and causing bruising. Significant bleeding and bruising of the forehead is important to avoid as it can often lead to the blood draining down to the tear trough area causing a bruised appearance under the eye which would be highly undesirable for the patient and prolonged their down time.
9. If any vessels are visible where the insertion site holes would be placed slightly shift the insertion site.

© The Author(s), under exclusive license to Springer Nature Switzerland AG 2023

N. M. Kim, *Non-Surgical Thread Procedures*, https://doi.org/10.1007/978-3-031-36468-6_11

Fig. 11.1 Pattern of thread insertion for lateral eyebrow lifting and lateral inferior crows

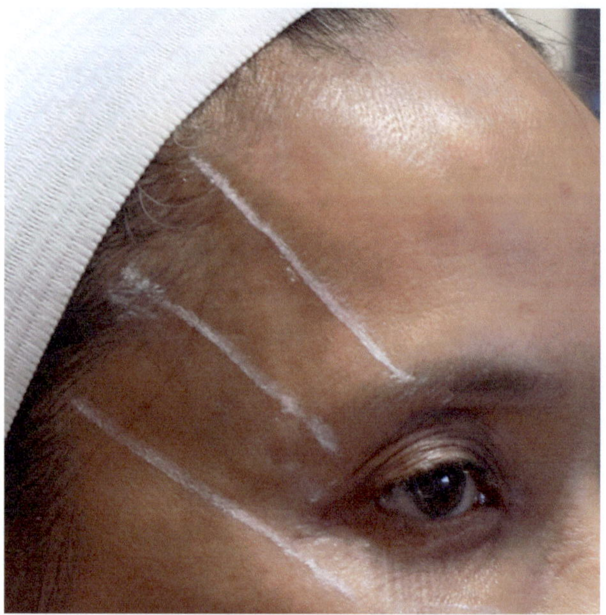

Fig. 11.2 Pattern of thread insertion for eyebrows and forehead lifting

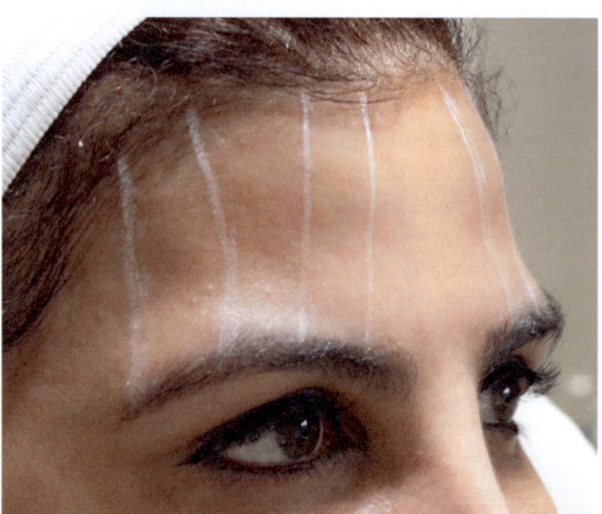

10. Make a wheal using the 30 g needle with the anesthetic at the insertion sites.
11. Using an 18-gauge needle make the pilot holes for the insertion sites.
12. Start on one side and proceed to the other and anesthetize each pathway using either a 23-, 25- or 27-gauge cannula depending on the patient's skin thickness. The cannula should be of 60-mm length.
13. Once the areas are anesthetized, begin inserting the threads with cannula. Start on one side and proceed to the other side.

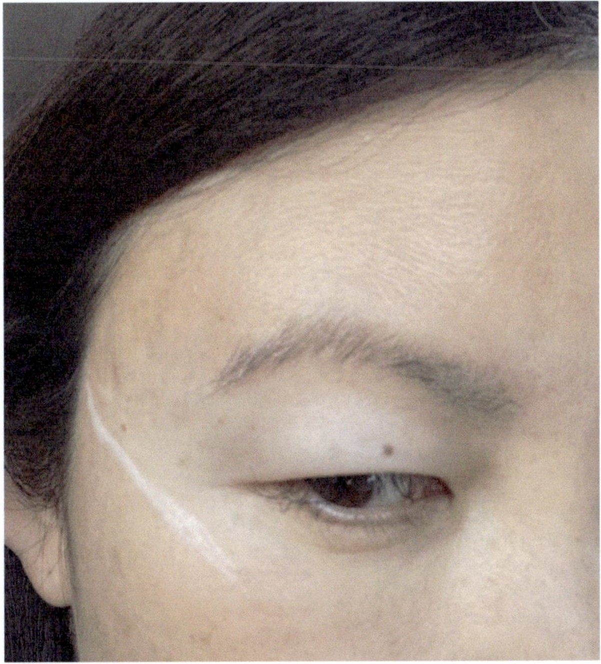

Fig. 11.3 Pattern of thread insertion for lateral inferior crow's feet and/or sagging skin in this area

14. When inserting the thread proceed slowly in order to avoid tearing vessels. Advance the cannula with thread as far as possible to include the entire length of the cannula. It is helpful to advance to tissue under the eyebrow and in fact slightly into the eyelid itself to get optimal results in terms of lifting.
15. Insert all the threads without tightening or lifting initially.
16. Once all the threads have been inserted begin to tighten gradually one at a time to get lift. It is helpful to lift as much as possible because ultimately the threads will relax and some of the lift will be lost.
17. Raise the patient to sitting position in order to reassess.
18. If any area needs more lifting do so while patient is in sitting position. If even after lifting as much as possible symmetry cannot be achieved and it appears that there is an area that needs more lifting draw another line in the area that is less lifted and add another thread. Be sure to place patient in supine position to insert any additional threads.
19. Once the lift is satisfactory, cut the threads one by one. Ensure that the cut is placed down low on the skin as much as possible so that the end of the thread is not protruding out of the skin. One can check this by placing your finger at the insertion site. If a sharp end of thread is still felt, then attempt to cut it more. If this is not possible, then attempt to massage the skin to cover the end of the thread.
20. Place antibiotic ointment on each of the thread insertion sites.

21. Figure 11.4 shows a photo of how the forehead may appear after the threads are placed. Be sure to reassure the patient that this swelling will go away as well as the excessive lift that may cause a surprised appearance. Generally, this will take 2–3 days. Of course, some patients may be perfectly happy with the excessive lift.

22. Advise patients to be gentle with this area, to avoid massage or significant rubbing while cleansing or while washing hair. Tenderness in this area for 5–7 days is normal.

23. Figure 11.5 shows photos of forehead at different stages after the procedure. Note that there remains slight irregularity of the skin which may occur depending on the age of the patient. However, this also will resolve in another 1–2 weeks in most patients.

24. Prescribe prophylactic antibiotics for 1 week. Recommend minocycline 100 mg bid for 7 days.

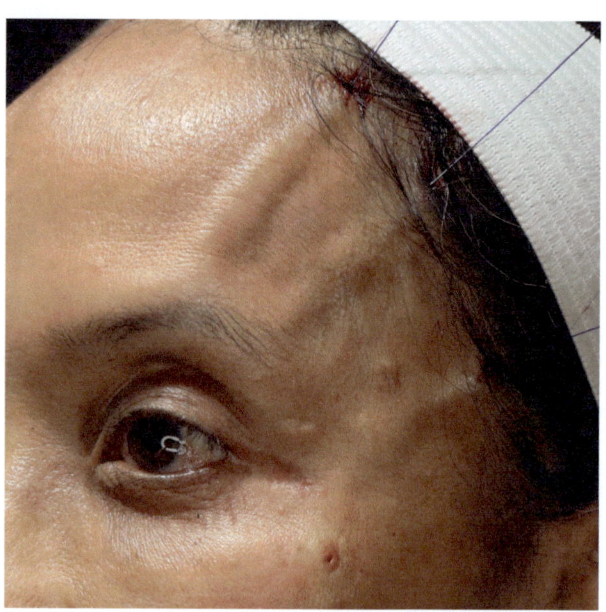

Fig. 11.4 Appearance of forehead immediately after thread lift eyebrows showing swelling that is normal

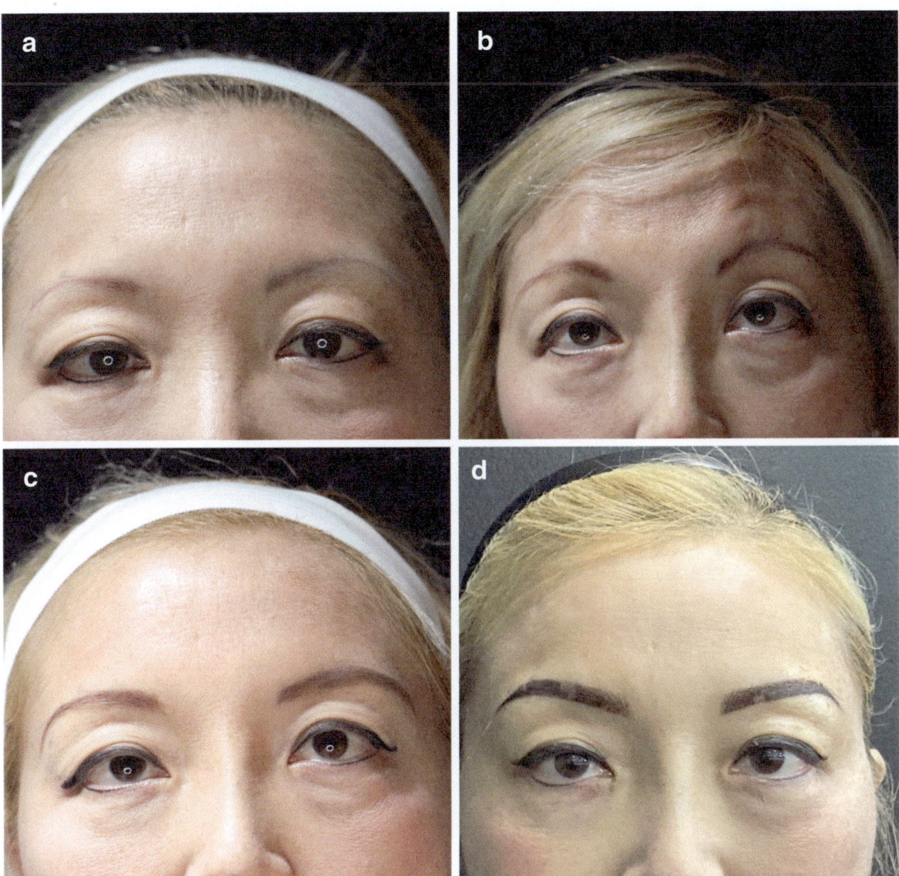

Fig. 11.5 Progression of Eyebrows and Forehead at different stages with treatment with barbed threads. (**a**) Immediately before treatment. (**b**) Immediately after treatment. (**c**) 3 weeks after treatment. (**d**) 6 weeks after treatment

Chapter 12
Procedure for Neck Lift with Barbed Threads

1. Remove makeup and cleanse the submental neck region with antiseptic cleanser.
2. Draw a line along the midline from the chin across the submental region (see Fig. 12.1). Draw additional lines perpendicularly to this line to correspond to the placement of the threads. Here 4 lines are drawn to correspond to 8 threads to be placed (4 threads on each side).
3. Use the white cosmetic pencil and the ruler to draw a line from this midline laterally under the mandible to the region below the earlobe measuring the length of the cannula. Draw additional lines as needed to cover the sagging region (see Instructional Video 33.1 in Chap. 33). At least two threads on each side are necessary; however, more threads may be needed for severe laxity.
4. Figure 12.2 shows the pattern of thread placement for severe laxity in the submental region using four barbed threads for each side so a total of 8 threads will be utilized.
5. Figure 12.3 also shows a pattern for thread placement for moderate laxity in a thinner patient in the submental region also using 4 threads on each side. It is helpful to be generous with the number of threads for the neck as it is a more challenging area for improvement compared to the face. Generally a total of 6-8 threads is recommended for most patients.
6. Place the patient in the supine position.
7. At the planned insertion sites make a wheal with the 2% lidocaine with epinephrine.
8. Use an 18-gauge needle to make the pilot holes.
9. Using a 22-gauge 100-mm cannula inject anesthetic along each pathway for the threads as drawn.
10. May anesthetize one side first and then insert the threads on the anesthetized side of the neck before proceeding to anesthetize the other side of the neck and then placing the threads on the other side.

© The Author(s), under exclusive license to Springer Nature Switzerland AG 2023

N. M. Kim, *Non-Surgical Thread Procedures*,
https://doi.org/10.1007/978-3-031-36468-6_12

Fig. 12.1 Thread placement pattern showing midline for severe laxity in submental region using eight barbed threads

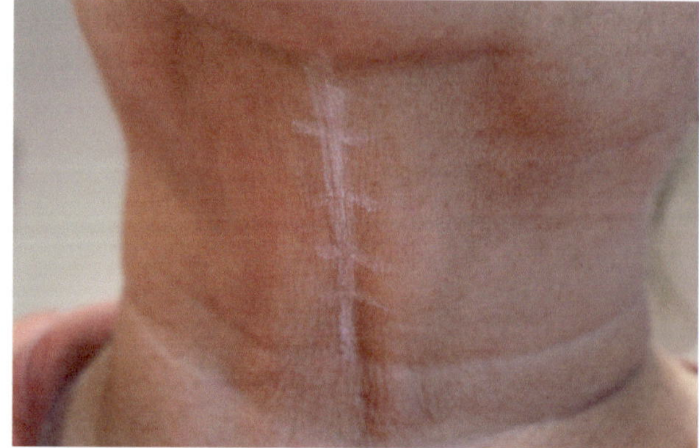

Fig. 12.2 Thread placement pattern for severe laxity in submental region using four barbed threads on each side

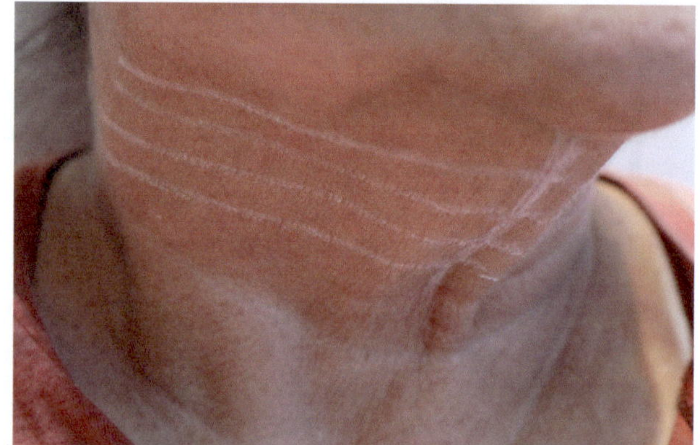

Fig. 12.3 Thread placement pattern for moderate laxity in submental region using four barbed threads for each side

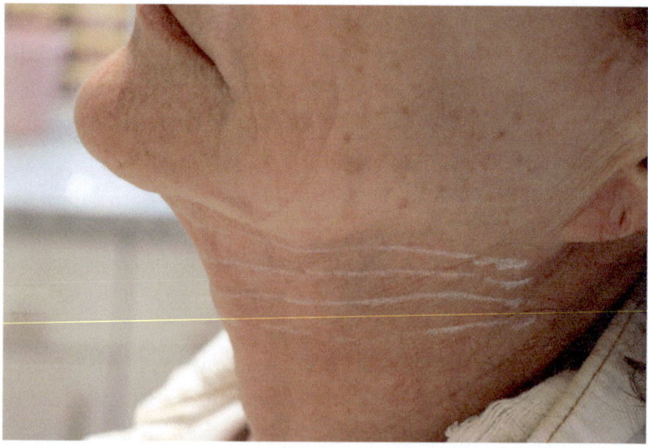

11. Once the thread pattern pathways are anesthetized on one side, may proceed to inserting the threads on the anesthetized side. The anesthesia is almost immediately effective so it is possible to proceed with inserting the threads almost immediately after anesthesia injection.
12. Start with the pathway closest to the mandible and work your way down the neck.
13. It is recommended to use Resculpt Medical Threads 18-gauge 100 mm barbed or cog thread for the neck. Since the neck is a challenging area, it is best to maximize improvement by using 18-gauge threads which are the strongest thickest thread. Since the area is generally hidden under the mandible, it is a forgiving area and using the thickest thread is tolerable. There will be less risk of breakage of thread with thicker threads and more collagen stimulation.
14. Be sure to insert the thread all the way to the midline point. Also, insert all the threads on both sides without tightening at first.
15. For threads that are lower on the neck, it is helpful to put a slight bend or curve on the cannula by bending it manually (see Fig.10.2). This allows you to follow the curve of the neck when inserting the thread so that it is easier to reach the midline (see Instructional Videos 33.2 and 33.3 in Chap. 33).
16. Once all the threads have been inserted on both sides then the tightening can begin.
17. Grab one thread that is at the same level on each side at the same time with each hand. Simultaneously pull on both sides and push the skin down towards the pulling end to tighten the skin. Do the same procedure with the next set of threads (see Instructional Video 33.3 in Chap. 33). This ensures that one side is not significantly pulled tighter than the other side allowing for improvement equally on both sides. If one side is pulled initially before the other side, it is not possible to pull the second side as tight.
18. Once all threads have been tightened and tissues approximated then raise the patient into the sitting position. Reassess the patient from the front and from the side checking for symmetry. If one side needs to be pulled tighter, do so at this time. If any thread needs to be pulled tighter, this can be done at this time as well with the patient supine. One does not have to worry as much about any significant dimpling as it is generally not visible in this area and will resolve. If, however, there is significant dimpling and bunching at the lateral aspect near the insertion sites, it is recommended to loosen slightly since too much buckling will require a prolonged period to resolve.
19. Once the threads placement and tightness are satisfactory, proceed to cut the threads.
20. Be sure to cut the thread down low on the skin as much as possible by pushing down with the iris scissors on the skin while cutting (see Instructional Video 33.3 in Chap. 33). Check that there is no end of thread left by feeling the insertion hole for any sharpness. If any remains, try to cut again or massage the skin over the end of the thread and encourage it to be buried. Once all the threads are cut apply antibiotic ointment to the insertion holes.

21. Prescribe prophylactic antibiotics for 1 week. Recommend Minocycline 100 mg twice a day.
22. Be sure to remind the patient to avoid exertional activity requiring significant rotation of the head for the next 1–2 weeks depending on discomfort. Also advise the patient to eat only soft foods as chewing will also be affected and painful during the first week after the procedure.
23. Figures 12.4, 12.5, and 12.6 show the photos of the appearance before and immediately after threads placement in the same patient.

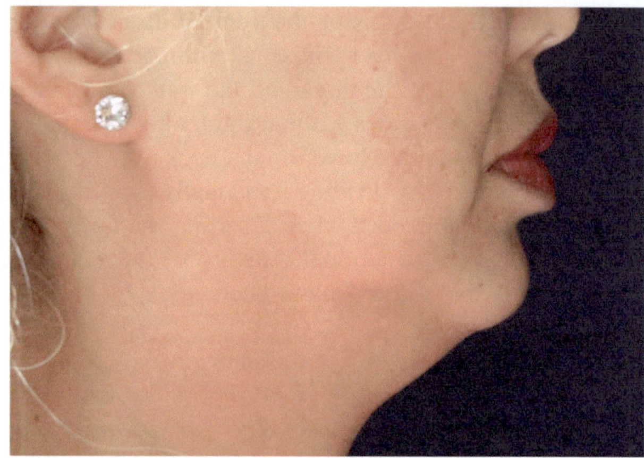

Fig. 12.4 Submental neck with moderate laxity in young patient before procedure

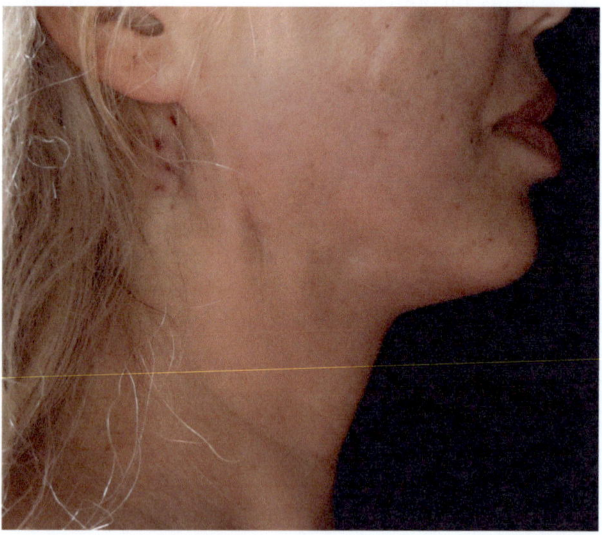

Fig. 12.5 Neck immediately after procedure with four barbed threads in the same patient shown in Fig. 12.4

Fig. 12.6 Submental Neck 1 month after procedure in the same patient shown in Fig. 12.5

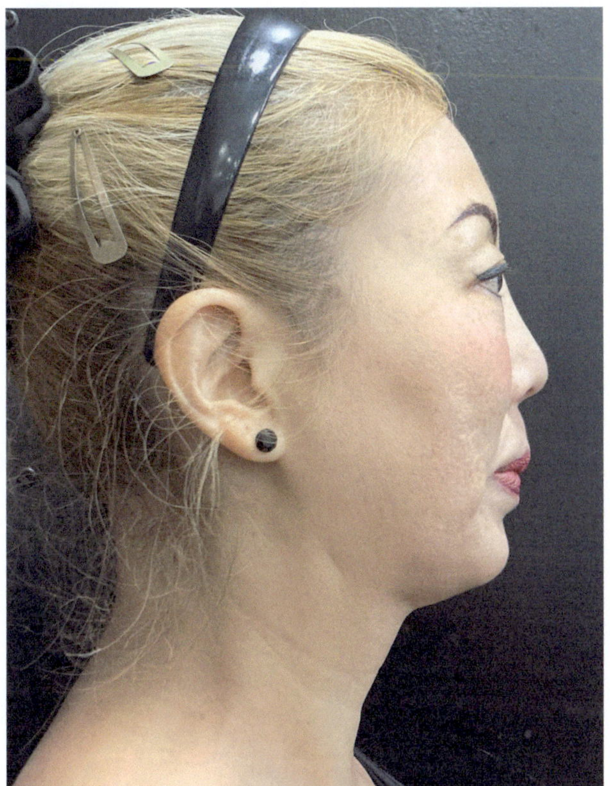

Chapter 13
Procedure for Browbone Building with Mesh Thread

1. Cleanse the eyebrow region with anti-septic cleanser.
2. Draw with white cosmetic pencil a line from the lateral end of the eyebrow to the medial third of the eyebrow (see Fig. 13.1).
3. Using a 30 g needle, inject a small amount of the anesthetic 2% Lidocaine with Epinephrine until you see a wheal at the lateral end which will be the entry site.
4. Make a pilot entry hole with an 18G needle at the site of this wheal.
5. Using a 23 or 25 g cannula of 50 or 60 mm length, enter through the pilot hole and anesthetize the path from the hole under the eyebrow to approximately 4 cm medially across the eyebrow.
6. Repeat anesthesia for the other eyebrow in the same manner.
7. Once anesthesia is completed, insert one Resculpt Medical Thread 19 g × 38 mm mesh Boost thread through the pilot hole and advance under the skin subcutaneously until the entire length of the cannula is under the skin. It is often helpful to advance even slightly further to ensure that the thread end remains inside the skin after cannula removal.
8. Remove the cannula while putting slight pressure on the distal end to encourage the engagement of the thread so that it will remain in place under the skin while the cannula is being removed.
9. Repeat for the other side.
10. Apply antibiotic ointment to the holes.
11. Advise the patient that final results will be seen after 2 months although some immediate change is visible as well. Figure 13.2 shows an example of the change in contour of browbone before and 2 months after the mesh procedure. Note that eyebrows appear more elevated in addition to reduction of thin, flat contour.

© The Author(s), under exclusive license to Springer Nature Switzerland AG 2023

N. M. Kim, *Non-Surgical Thread Procedures*,
https://doi.org/10.1007/978-3-031-36468-6_13

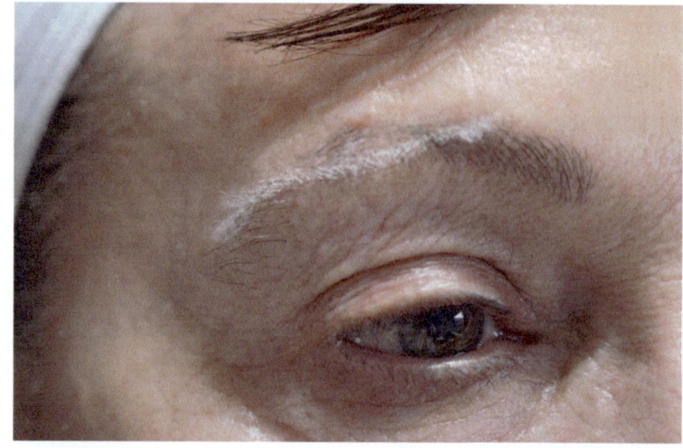

Fig. 13.1 Drawing of pathway of the thread for browbone building with mesh thread

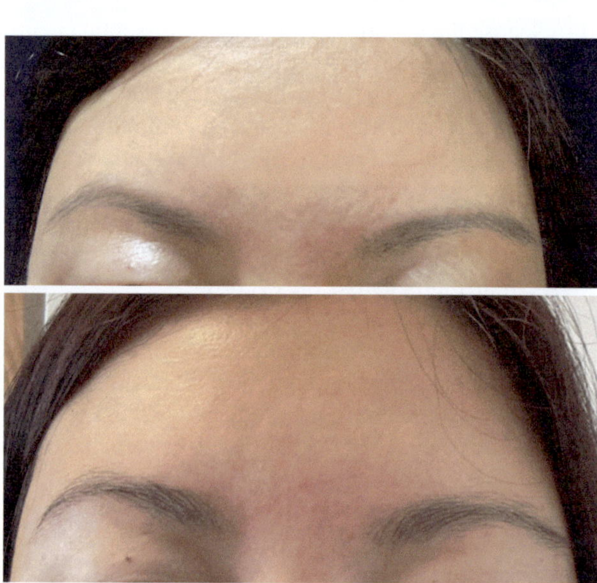

Fig. 13.2 Before and after mesh threads treatment for browbones

Chapter 14
Procedure for Treatment of Undereye Hollows and Anterior Cheeks with Mesh Threads

1. Remove makeup and cleanse the area with alcohol or antiseptic cleanser.
2. Using a flexible ruler and a white cosmetic pencil mark two lines under each tear troughs region. Use the ruler to measure 4 cm for the length of the line. It is possible to enter slightly within the area of the tear trough or to stay just outside of the edge. Have the two lines cross any indentation that the patient may have extending from the tear trough. The two lines may be between half centimeter to 1 cm apart (See Fig. 14.1 and Instructional Video 33.1. in Chap. 33).
3. Make a wheal with the anesthetic 2% Lidocaine with Epinephrine at the lateral end of each line.
4. Using an 18-gauge needle make pilot holes at each entry site.
5. Using a 23- or 25-gauge cannula of 38 or greater millimeter length enter through the pilot holes and anesthetize along each line of planned thread.
6. Once all the paths are anesthetized, proceed to insert the threads. It is recommended to use Resculpt Medical Threads that are 19 gauge by 38-mm length mesh Boost threads. Enter through the insertion site and advance gradually. If resistance is met, retract and redirect deeper and use a rotating or twisting motion on the cannula to help ease of entry. It is also helpful to try to drape the skin over the cannula using the other hand. Insert to the entire length of the cannula and slightly further if possible.
7. When removing the cannula apply pressure at the distal end with your other hand to try to engage the thread to stay inside the skin (See Instructional Video 33.2 in Chap.33). If the thread does not stay inside the skin entirely, then it must be removed and insertion attempted again with a brand new thread.
8. Repeat the insertion technique for all threads.
9. Once all the threads are inserted apply antibiotic ointment to the entry hole sites.
10. Instruct the patient that full effect from the treatment will be seen in 2 months although some immediate effect will also be apparent. Figures 14.2 and 14.3 show the before and after 2 months improvement in hollowing of undereye region.

© The Author(s), under exclusive license to Springer Nature Switzerland AG 2023

N. M. Kim, *Non-Surgical Thread Procedures*, https://doi.org/10.1007/978-3-031-36468-6_14

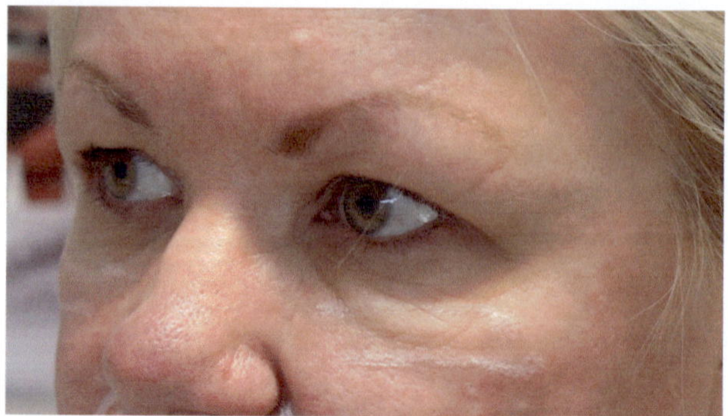

Fig. 14.1 Lines drawn showing pattern of mesh thread insertion in tear trough region

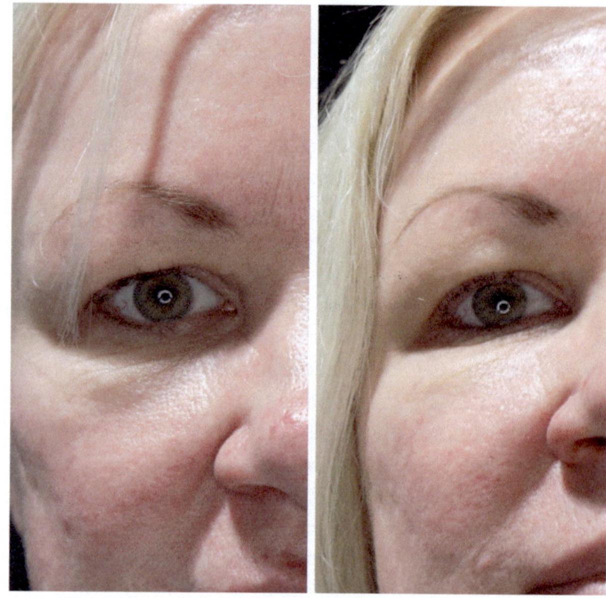

Fig. 14.2 Before and 2 months after mesh thread placement in tear trough region

Fig. 14.3 Before and 2 months after mesh thread placement in undereye region

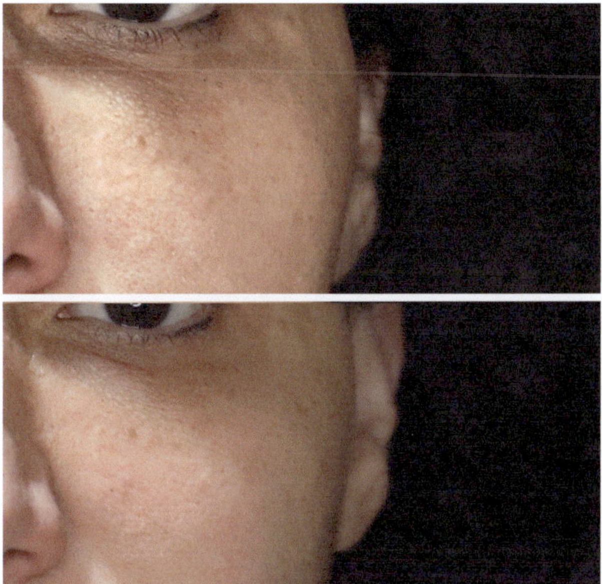

Chapter 15
Procedure for Treatment of Nasolabial Fold with Mesh Threads

1. Remove makeup and cleanse the nasolabial fold area with alcohol or antiseptic cleanser.
2. Using a flexible ruler and white cosmetic pencil draw two lines each 4 cm long along the nasolabial fold as shown in Fig. 15.1 and Instructional Video 33.1 in Chap.33. This pattern allows for use of only a single insertion hole for two threads on each side.
3. Using the 30-gauge needle make a wheal with the anesthetic (2% lidocaine with epinephrine) at the inferior end of the line.
4. Make an entry hole at the site of the wheal with the 18-gauge needle.
5. Using a 23-gauge or 25-gauge cannula with the length of between 38 mm and 60 mm enter through the insertion hole and anesthetize the pathway drawn for the threads. Once both sides are anesthetized proceed to insert the threads.
6. It is recommended to use Resculpt Medical Threads that are 19 gauge 38-mm mesh Boost threads. Enter through the insertion hole while stretching the skin with your other hand. It is helpful to rotate or twist the thread back and forth to ease entry rather than simply pushing. Be patient as the cannula will eventually be able to be inserted along its entire length if one proceeds with a gentle methodical manner. It is also helpful to insert the cannula and drape the skin over it with your other hand to cover the thread. See Instructional Video 33.2 in Chap. 33 for a demonstration of this procedure.
7. Once the thread is inserted entirely, use your other hand to place slight pressure at the distal end of the thread and cannula. While rotating the cannula back and forth remove the cannula slowly. You may feel a slight click or hear a slight click as the thread is released out of the cannula and is held within the skin. This is ideal for when the cannula is fully removed, the thread should be entirely under the skin without any protruding end. If there is a protruding end outside of the entry hole, unfortunately the entire thread will need to be removed and the procedure will have to be attempted again with a brand-new thread. Once all the threads are inserted in this manner then place antibiotic ointment on the holes.

© The Author(s), under exclusive license to Springer Nature
Switzerland AG 2023
N. M. Kim, *Non-Surgical Thread Procedures*,
https://doi.org/10.1007/978-3-031-36468-6_15

Fig. 15.1 Pattern of mesh thread insertion for nasolabial folds

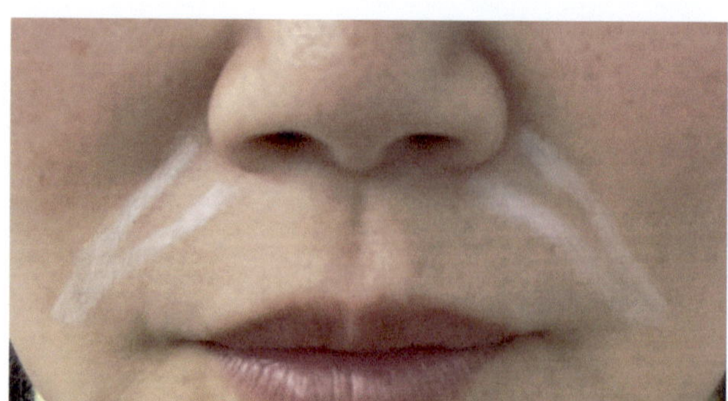

Chapter 16
Procedure for Treatment of Marionette Lines with Mesh Threads

1. Remove makeup and cleanse the area with alcohol or other antiseptic cleanser.
2. With white cosmetic pencil and flexible ruler draw lines crossing the marionette line of either 4 cm or 6 cm depending on whether chin is to be included. See Figs. 16.1 and 16.2 for different patterns.
3. Inject a wheal of anesthesia (2% Lidocaine with Epinephrine) at the entry sites. If only treating the marionette line alone, entry sites can be more lateral on the face. If treating the chin as well one can use a single medial insertion site on the chin.
4. Using an 18-gauge needle make the entry holes at the sites desired. Using a 60-mm 23 gauge or 25-gauge cannula enter through the insertion site and anesthetize the pathway marked by the lines drawn.
5. Once fully anesthetized proceed with inserting the threads.
6. It is recommended to use Resculpt Medical Threads 19-gauge 38 mm or 60 mm mesh Boost threads depending on the size of area to be treated. Insert the cannula with thread through the entry hole. It is helpful to rotate the cannula with thread clockwise and counterclockwise to overcome any resistance. Also try to stretch the skin out smoothly with your other hand to make a smoother pathway of tissue to pass through. One can also try to drape the skin over the thread cannula as well to ease entry. These techniques are most easily learned by watching a demonstration and then being guided by a trainer in person.
7. Be sure to insert the thread and cannula completely along its length and slightly beyond by attempting to drape the skin over the cannula as much as possible. This is to ensure that the thread stays inside the tissue completely while the cannula is being withdrawn. If any part of the thread is protruding out of the skin, it is best to pull it out completely and start with a brand-new thread.
8. Once all threads are inserted, apply antibiotic ointment to the insertion holes.

© The Author(s), under exclusive license to Springer Nature Switzerland AG 2023

N. M. Kim, *Non-Surgical Thread Procedures*, https://doi.org/10.1007/978-3-031-36468-6_16

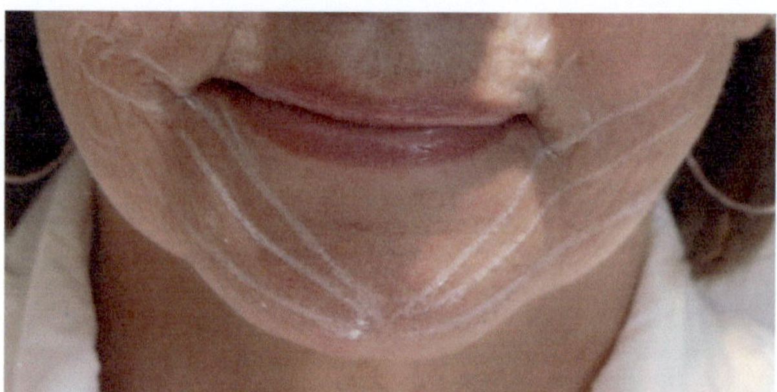

Fig. 16.1 Pattern of thread insertion for treatment of marionette lines with inclusion of chin

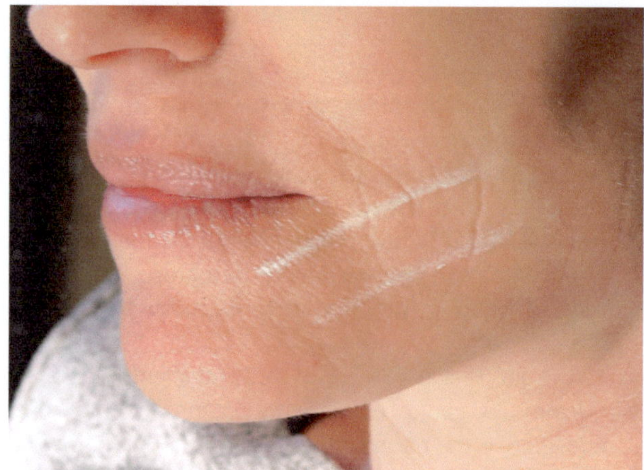

Fig. 16.2 Pattern of thread insertion for treatment of marionette lines without inclusion of chin

Chapter 17
Procedure for Treatment of Chin with Mesh Threads

1. Remove makeup and cleanse the area with alcohol or other antiseptic cleanser.
2. With a white cosmetic pencil and flexible ruler draw lines as shown in Fig. 17.1. The lines should be 4 cm in length.
3. Make a wheal of anesthetic (2% Lidocaine with Epinephrine) at the insertion site on the chin where lines converge.
4. Using an 18-gauge needle puncture the skin to make the insertion hole.
5. Using a 23- or 25-gauge cannula of between 38- and 60-mm length enter through the entry hole and anesthetize the pathway marked by the lines drawn.
6. Once all the pathways are anesthetized proceed with inserting the threads. It is recommended to use Resculpt Medical Threads that are 19-gauge 38-mm mesh Boost threads on cannula. Enter through the insertion site for each pathway. It is helpful to rotate the thread on cannula counterclockwise and clockwise to aid in overcoming any resistance of tissue. It is also helpful to stretch the skin with your other hand to provide a smoother pathway for the cannula to pass.
7. Insert the cannula as far as possible by draping some excess skin over the cannula. This is helpful in ensuring that the thread completely remains inside the tissue while the cannula is being withdrawn. If any of the thread is protruding out of the skin after the cannula is withdrawn, the entire thread must be taken out and a new thread must be reinserted.
8. Once all the threads have been inserted apply antibiotic appointment to the insertion sites.

© The Author(s), under exclusive license to Springer Nature Switzerland AG 2023
N. M. Kim, *Non-Surgical Thread Procedures*,
https://doi.org/10.1007/978-3-031-36468-6_17

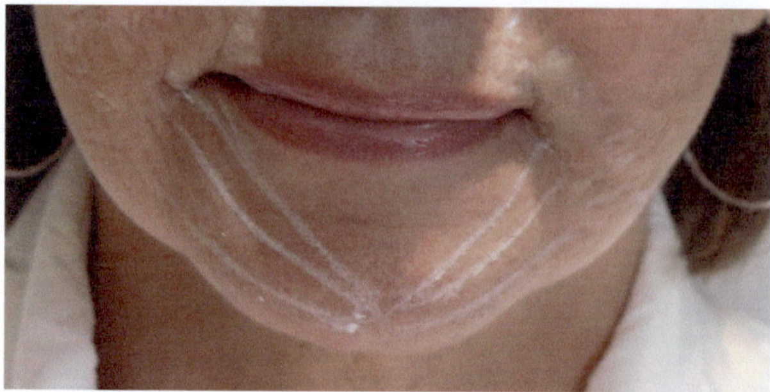

Fig. 17.1 Lines drawn representing pattern of threads for chin treatment with mesh threads

Chapter 18
Procedure for Treatment of Décolleté with Mesh Threads

1. Cleanse the area with alcohol or other antiseptic cleanser.
2. Draw lines of 4 cm in length down the midline of the décolleté. If needed, add some laterally in the upper region as well. See Fig. 18.1 for recommended pattern of insertion.
3. Inject a wheal of anesthesia (2% Lidocaine with Epinephrine) at the insertion sites located at one end of each line.
4. Using an 18-gauge needle puncture the skin at the insertion sites to make the entry holes.
5. Using a 23-gauge cannula of between 38 and 60 mm length, enter through the insertion holes and inject anesthesia along the entire pathway of the lines.
6. Once anesthesia is completed proceed with inserting the threads.
7. It is recommended to use Resculpt Medical Threads that are 19-gauge 38 mm length mesh Boost threads. Enter through the insertion holes and use a rotating motion to ease passage of the cannula with thread. Be sure to advance the cannula on thread as far as possible to ensure that the thread remains under the skin once the cannulas are retracted. Use the other hand to engage the end of thread that is under the skin while retracting the cannula. As with all mesh threads, if the thread is not completely buried under the skin after the cannula is retracted, remove the thread entirely and repeat the insertion with a new thread.
8. Once all the threads are inserted apply antibiotic ointment to the insertion holes.

© The Author(s), under exclusive license to Springer Nature Switzerland AG 2023
N. M. Kim, *Non-Surgical Thread Procedures*,
https://doi.org/10.1007/978-3-031-36468-6_18

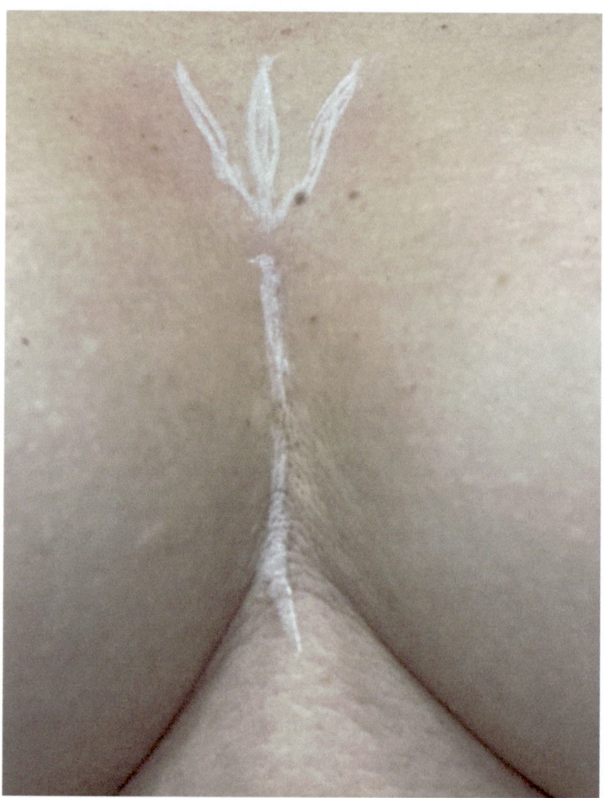

Fig. 18.1 Pattern of thread insertion for treatment of décolleté with mesh threads

Chapter 19
Procedure for Treatment of Thin Crepey Skin with Mesh Threads

1. Remove makeup and cleanse the area with alcohol or antiseptic cleanser.
2. Using a white cosmetic pencil and flexible ruler draw lines with corresponding length of the thread you plan to use across the region of thin crepey skin. The lines should be either 4 cm for smaller areas or 6 cm for larger areas. See Fig. 19.1 for an example of lines drawn through crepey skin of an upper cheek area. The lines should be no more than 1 cm apart and as close as 3 mm close to each other.
3. Make a wheal with 2% lidocaine with epinephrine at the entry sites. It is preferable to have the entry sites be at the most lateral end of the thread pathway.
4. Using an 18-gauge needle, puncture the skin to make the insertion holes for each line.
5. Using a 23- or 25-gauge cannula of between 38 and 60 mm in length, anesthetize each pathway indicated by the lines drawn. Once all the pathways are anesthetized, proceed with the insertion of the threads on cannula.
6. It is recommended to use Resculpt Medical Threads that are 19-gauge 38-mm length or 19-gauge 60-mm length mesh Boost threads depending on the dimensions of the area requiring correction. Insert the thread on cannula through the insertion holes. Rotating the thread and cannula clockwise and counterclockwise aids in overcoming resistance and is preferred over pushing too forcefully. It is important to have patience during the insertion. Using the left hand (for right handers) to stretch the skin out can also create a smoother pathway for the thread insertion. The left hand can also be used to drape the skin over the cannula rather than pushing the cannula forcefully. These maneuvers aid in making insertion a gentler careful process.
7. Insert all the threads. Ensure that no end of thread is protruding out of the skin after the cannulas are retracted. If end of thread protrudes, remove the thread altogether and insert with a brand-new thread. Apply antibiotic ointment to all insertion holes.

© The Author(s), under exclusive license to Springer Nature
Switzerland AG 2023
N. M. Kim, *Non-Surgical Thread Procedures*,
https://doi.org/10.1007/978-3-031-36468-6_19

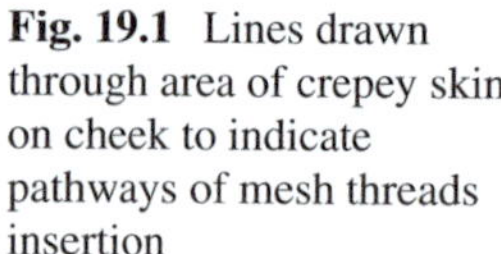

Fig. 19.1 Lines drawn through area of crepey skin on cheek to indicate pathways of mesh threads insertion

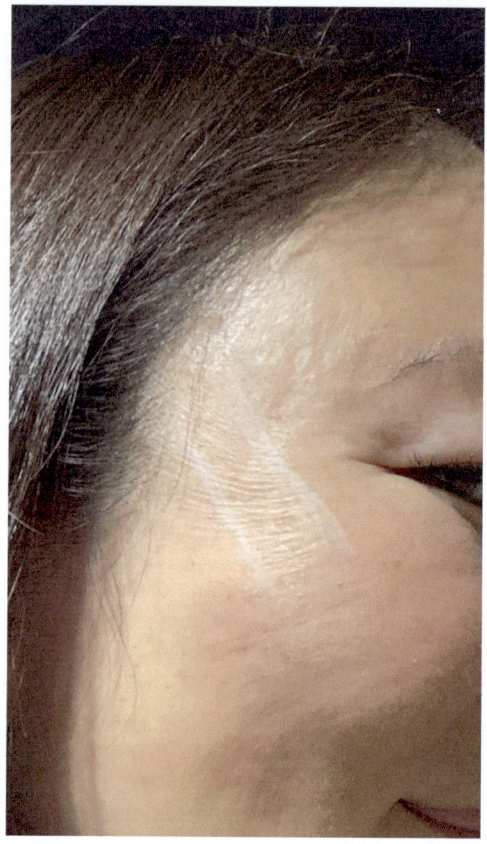

Chapter 20
Procedure for Treatment of Cheeks with Mono Threads

1. Remove makeup and cleanse the area with alcohol or other antiseptic cleanser.
2. Using a white cosmetic pencil and flexible ruler draw lines for the pathway of the threads to be inserted. Draw the lines in a mesh pattern if possible. Draw the length of the lines according to the length of the threads to be used in the area to be covered. See Fig. 20.1.
3. Use enough threads to cover the area in a mesh pattern with spacing approximately 0.5 cm between the threads.
4. For the cheeks it is preferable to use Resculpt Medical Threads that are 27-gauge 38-mm length mono threads and to use at least 10 threads on each side. Larger gauge such as 25 or 23 gauge may be used as well if skin is thick enough. On thin skin use thinner gauge threads but more of them.
5. Decide on a point of insertion of a cannula that will allow for anesthesia to be easily injected to anesthetize the entire region. Make a wheal with 2% lidocaine and epinephrine using a 30-gauge needle and syringe. Make the entry hole with a 22-gauge needle. Then use a 25-gauge cannula to inject the anesthesia into the area.
6. Mono threads to be used will be loaded on needles so it is not necessary to make pilot holes prior to insertion if the mono threads are of thin gauge. However, for thicker mono threads such as 23 g, pilot holes may need to be made especially if the threads are longer than 50 mm. Insert the threads along the lines drawn. Entry in the lateral areas of the face is preferred as any bruising will be in the less visible areas of the face that can be covered with hair. Bruising is possible since the threads are on needles with this procedure.
7. When inserting the threads be sure to insert deeply enough so that you are in the subcutaneous tissue not in the dermis.
8. If inserting the thread along a curved bone contouring is possible by using your other hand to put some pressure in order to keep a bend in the thread along the curve through the skin. The needles are fairly flexible and allow for this in order to keep the needle at the proper depth of the skin.

© The Author(s), under exclusive license to Springer Nature
Switzerland AG 2023
N. M. Kim, *Non-Surgical Thread Procedures*,
https://doi.org/10.1007/978-3-031-36468-6_20

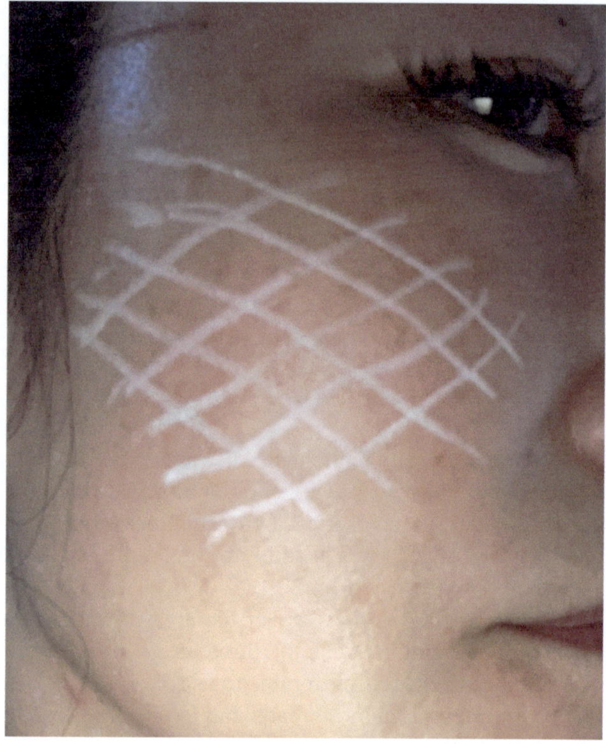

Fig. 20.1 Lines drawn to indicate pattern of mono threads to be inserted for treatment of cheeks skin

9. it is possible to either insert a single thread and remove the needle for that thread and proceed this way one at a time or to insert several threads at once leaving the needles in the skin initially and then removing all or several needles at one time.
10. Once all the threads are inserted apply antibiotic ointment to the area for faster healing. Also apply pressure to decrease any bleeding and minimize bruising.

Chapter 21
Procedure for Treatment of Jowls with Mono Threads

1. Remove makeup and cleanse the area to be treated with alcohol or antiseptic cleanser.
2. Draw lines with the white cosmetic pencil as shown in Fig. 21.1. Draw lines in a mesh pattern with approximately 5 mm between the lines. It is recommended to use Resculpt Medical Threads that are 27-Gauge 38-mm mono threads or 27-Gauge 50-mm mono threads depending on the size of the patients face and jowls area. Thus, the lines should be drawn of corresponding length. Thicker gauge threads such as 25 or 23 G may be used if the patient has relatively thick skin.
3. Decide on a point of insertion of a cannula that will allow for anesthesia to be easily injected to anesthetize the entire region. Make a wheal at this location with 2% lidocaine with epinephrine using a 30 G needle and syringe. Then make the entry hole with a 22-G needle. Then use a 25-Gauge cannula of appropriate length to inject the anesthesia into the area.
4. Thin mono threads such as 27 Gauge will be loaded on needles so it is not necessary to make pilot holes for the threads. Thicker mono threads of 25 or 23 G will be more comfortable for the patient if pilot holes are made at anesthetized insertion sites. Insert the threads along the lines drawn. Entry in the periphery of the face is preferred as any bruising will be in the less visible portions of the face and may be covered by hair. Bruising is possible since the threads are on needles with this procedure.
5. When inserting the threads be sure to insert deeply enough so that you are in the subcutaneous tissue not in the dermis.
6. It is possible to either insert a single thread and remove the needle for that thread and proceed this way one at a time or to insert several threads at once leaving the needles in the skin initially and then removing all or the several needles at one time.
7. Once all the threads are inserted apply antibiotic ointment to the area for faster healing. Also apply pressure to decrease any bleeding and minimize bruising.

© The Author(s), under exclusive license to Springer Nature Switzerland AG 2023

N. M. Kim, *Non-Surgical Thread Procedures*,
https://doi.org/10.1007/978-3-031-36468-6_21

Fig. 21.1 Lines drawn
indicating pattern of
insertion for mono threads
in the jowl area

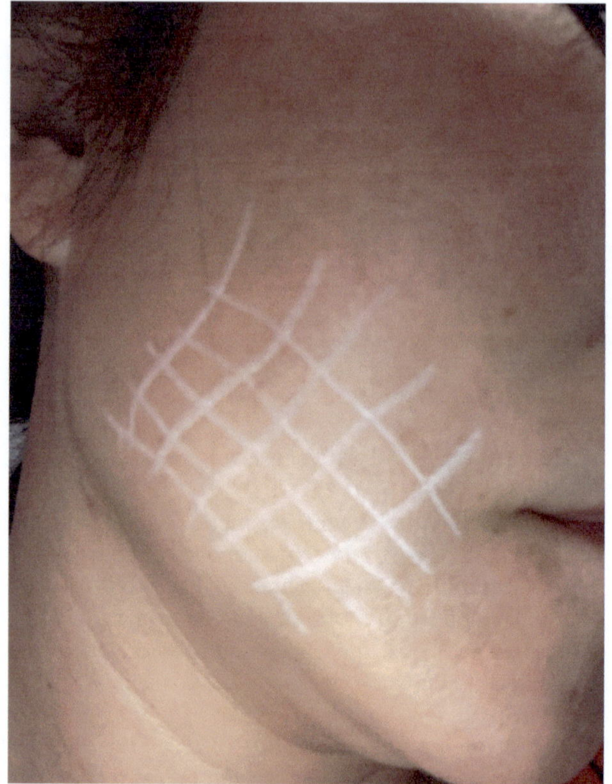

Chapter 22
Procedure for Treatment of Necklace Lines with Mono Threads

1. Remove makeup and cleanse the skin with alcohol or other antiseptic cleanser.
2. Apply numbing cream to the lines to be treated. Allow at least 20 min for the numbing cream to take effect. It is helpful to occlude the numbing cream by covering with plastic wrap. Once anesthesia has been achieved wipe off the numbing cream and clean with alcohol.
3. It is recommended to use Resculpt Medical Threads 25-G 38-mm length spring threads, however, smaller gauge thinner spring or mono threads can also be used, particularly if the patient is older or has thinner skin. A length of 50 mm may be used also, however, the 38 mm is easier to manage due to the curvature of the neck.
4. Starting from one side laterally, insert the thread directly into the necklace line. Make sure to be subcutaneous rather than too superficial otherwise the thread may be visible. It is helpful when inserting to stretch the skin or drape it over the thread. It may be helpful to either press with the other hand down through the skin onto the needle to bend it so that it follows along with the curve of the neck. Alternatively, one can tent up the skin to provide a flatter contour to ease passage of the thread.
5. Start the following thread where the previous thread ended in order to cover the line completely. It is helpful also to overlap especially in areas where the line may be particularly deep or wide. Insert one thread at a time and remove the needle immediately afterwards or do several at a time before removing the needles at once (see Fig. 22.1).
6. If any thread does not completely stay under the skin, then remove it and replace with a new one.
7. Continue to insert the threads one after another until all lines are treated. This may require 10 or more threads.
8. Once all threads are inserted apply antibiotic ointment to the insertion holes.

© The Author(s), under exclusive license to Springer Nature
Switzerland AG 2023

N. M. Kim, *Non-Surgical Thread Procedures*,
https://doi.org/10.1007/978-3-031-36468-6_22

Fig. 22.1 Resculpt
medical threads 25-G
38-mm PDO spring threads
inserted into necklace lines

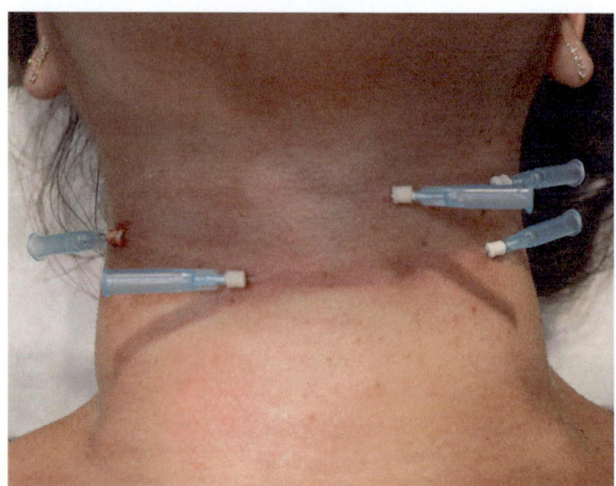

Chapter 23
Procedure for Treatment of Mild Submental Neck Laxity with Mono Threads

1. Anesthetize the submental skin with numbing cream. Allow at least 20 min for the numbing cream to take effect. It is helpful to occlude the cream onto the skin with plastic wrap as well. It may also be more comfortable for the patient if anesthetized with subcutaneous injections of 2% lidocaine with epinephrine particularly in the insertion sites.
2. Once the area is anaesthetized remove the numbing cream with alcohol and cleanse the area.
3. It is preferable to use Resculpt Medical Threads that are 27-G, 25-G, or 23-G 38-mm mono threads for this area. For thinner more lax skin, the thicker 23-G will produce better results.
4. Insert threads in the pattern as shown in Fig. 23.1. The more threads used, the better the result will be. Between 10 and 20 threads are recommended to be inserted.
5. Be sure to insert threads into the subcutaneous layer and not too superficially.
6. Once all the threads are inserted apply antibiotic ointment to the area.

© The Author(s), under exclusive license to Springer Nature Switzerland AG 2023
N. M. Kim, *Non-Surgical Thread Procedures*,
https://doi.org/10.1007/978-3-031-36468-6_23

Fig. 23.1 Lines drawn indicating pattern of mono thread placement for submental neck region

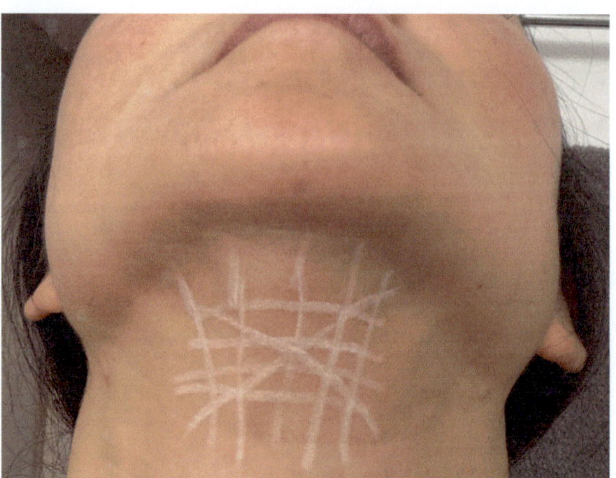

Chapter 24
Procedure for Treatment of Anterior Neck with Mono Threads

1. Apply numbing cream to the anterior neck area to be treated. Allow at least 20 min for the anesthesia to take effect. It is helpful to occlude the cream with plastic wrap on the skin as well. It may also be more comfortable for the patient to inject subcutaneously with 2% lidocaine with epinephrine through the area or at least at the sites where the threads will puncture the skin.
2. Once area is anesthetized, cleanse the area with alcohol.
3. It is recommended to use Resculpt Medical Threads that are 27, 25, or 23-Gauge 38 mm mono threads or 25 or 23-G 38 mm spring threads if significant laxity. Use thinner threads (higher gauge number) for thinner more lax skin. For example, if patient is thin and with thin skin, insert 27 Gauge or 25 Gauge threads. Reserve 23 Gauge threads for those with thicker skin and more fatty tissue. This will avoid the complication of irregularity of the skin due to thread being too superficial.
4. It is best to place the threads in a mesh pattern. See Fig. 24.1 for one option for the pattern of placement. The more threads that can be used the better the improvement. It may be necessary to use 20–30 threads or more depending on the size of the neck and area to be treated.
5. Insert the threads ensuring that the placement is subcutaneous and not too superficial. It is helpful to use the other hand to put pressure through the skin while inserting the thread into an area with curved contour. Place the threads as close to each other as possible. See Fig. 24.2.
6. Once all the threads are inserted apply antibiotic ointment to the area.

© The Author(s), under exclusive license to Springer Nature Switzerland AG 2023
N. M. Kim, *Non-Surgical Thread Procedures*,
https://doi.org/10.1007/978-3-031-36468-6_24

Fig. 24.1 Lines drawn showing the recommended pattern of insertion of mono threads in anterior neck region

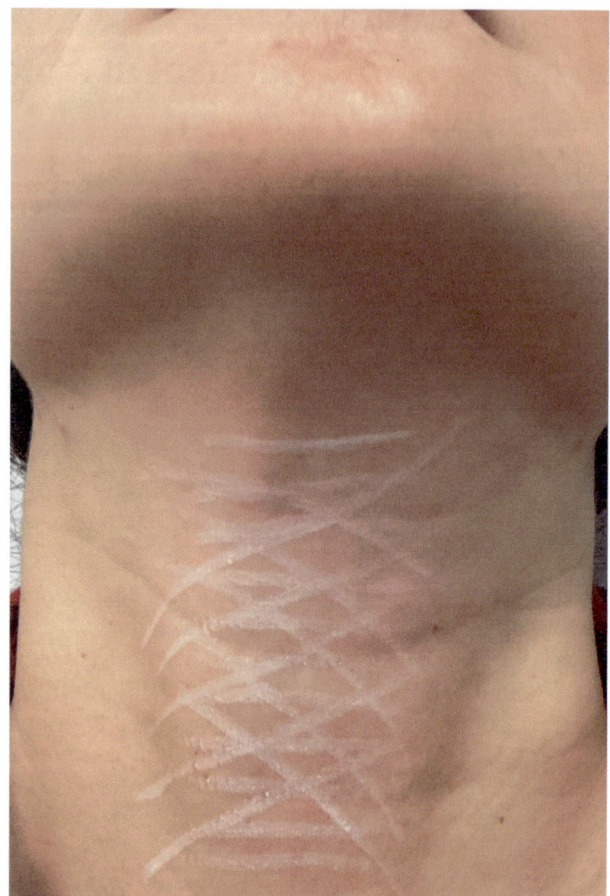

Fig. 24.2 Needle hubs showing placement of horizontal direction threads. Note the threads are inserted very close to each other in order to maximize the number of threads inserted and optimize collagen stimulation

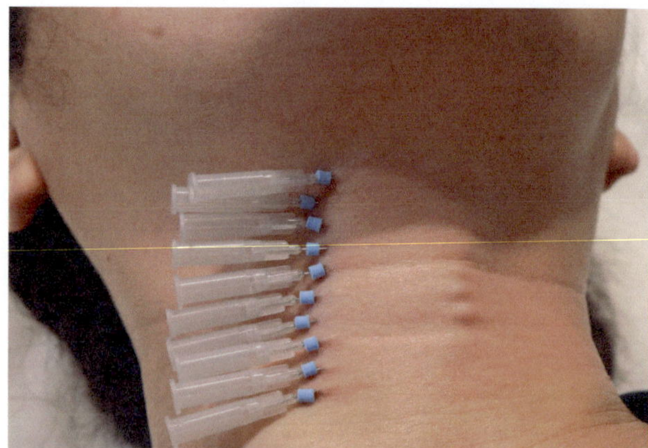

Chapter 25
Procedure for Treatment of Upper Arms

1. Cleanse the area with alcohol or other antiseptic cleanser.
2. Inject local anesthesia subcutaneously in the region to be treated with 2% lidocaine with epinephrine using either a 30 G needle or using a cannula after making a pilot hole. Choose the cannula length according to the area that is desired to be treated.
3. Insert threads in a mesh pattern. It is recommended to use Resculpt Medical Threads that are 25 Gauge or 23 Gauge mono threads and are 60 or 90 mm in length for the threads to be inserted vertically. Use 25- or 23-G mono threads that are 60 mm in length for the threads to be inserted horizontally. Choose the length of thread depending on the size of the patient's arms. See Figs. 25.1 and 25.2.
4. Even though the threads are loaded on sharp end cannulas, it is still necessary to create an entry hole for each thread with a 22 Gauge or 20 Gauge needle. The threads loaded on sharp cannulas that are 60 mm or 90 mm in length are still not stiff enough to puncture the skin easily.
5. It is best to have the threads be between 0.5 mm and 1 cm apart to ensure more uniform improvement. Use between 20 and 40 threads per arm for optimal results. The more threads used, the better the result will be.
6. Insert the threads ensuring that they are inserted subcutaneously and not too superficially. Be sure to make sure that all of the thread is buried under the skin. If there is any thread that is protruding out of the skin, it must be removed and replaced with a new thread.
7. Once all the threads have been inserted apply antibiotic ointment to the area.
8. Prescribe prophylactic antibiotics such as Minocycline 100 mg twice a day for 5 days.

© The Author(s), under exclusive license to Springer Nature
Switzerland AG 2023
N. M. Kim, *Non-Surgical Thread Procedures*,
https://doi.org/10.1007/978-3-031-36468-6_25

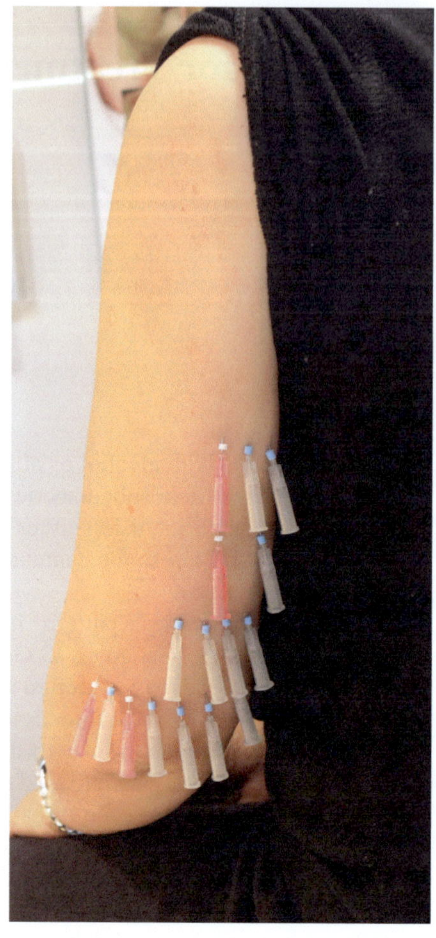

Fig. 25.1 Mono threads inserted vertically in posterior upper arms

Fig. 25.2 Mono threads inserted horizontally in posterior upper arms

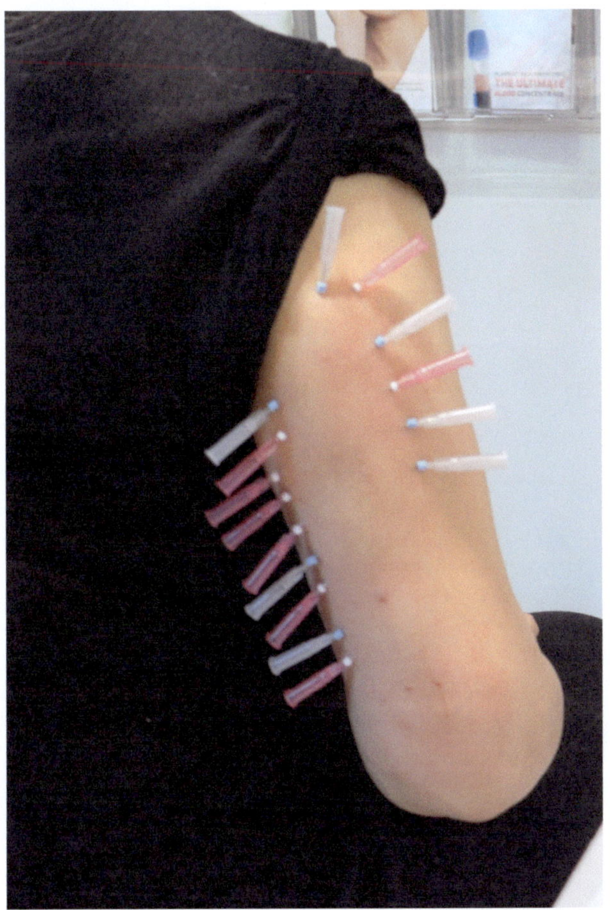

Chapter 26
Procedure for Treatment of Abdominal Skin

1. Cleanse the area to be treated with alcohol or other antiseptic cleanser.
2. Using a white cosmetic pencil and flexible ruler draw lines in a mesh pattern to plan the placement of the threads. Draw the lines according to the length of the threads to be inserted. Plan to use enough threads to have less than 1 cm of space between the threads. See Fig. 26.1.
3. It is recommended to use Resculpt Medical Threads that are 23 Gauge 60 mm or 90 mm length mono, spring or barbed threads depending on the size and condition of the skin to be treated. Select mono threads if moderately thin skin, spring threads if thin skin with more laxity needing thickening with collagen, and use barbed threads if need more fat reduction in thicker skin.
4. Inject local anesthesia subcutaneously in the entire region to be treated with 2% lidocaine with epinephrine using a cannula after creating a pilot hole with an 18 G needle at an anesthetized site. Choose the cannula length according to the area that is desired to be treated.
5. Insert the threads along the lines drawn for the pathways of the threads. Be sure to insert in the subcutaneous layer rather than dermal. Do not place too superficially.
6. Even though mono threads and spring threads will be loaded on sharp cannulas, it is still necessary to create entry holes with an 18 G needle for each thread. Due to the length of 60 mm or 90 mm cannulas, they are still not stiff enough and too unwieldy to puncture the skin easily. And of course, if using barbed threads which are usually loaded on blunt cannulas, an entry hole must always be made using an 18 needle as well.
7. Once all threads have been inserted apply antibiotic ointment to promote faster healing.
8. Prescribe prophylactic antibiotics such as Minocycline 100 mg twice a day for 7 days.

© The Author(s), under exclusive license to Springer Nature Switzerland AG 2023

N. M. Kim, *Non-Surgical Thread Procedures*,
https://doi.org/10.1007/978-3-031-36468-6_26

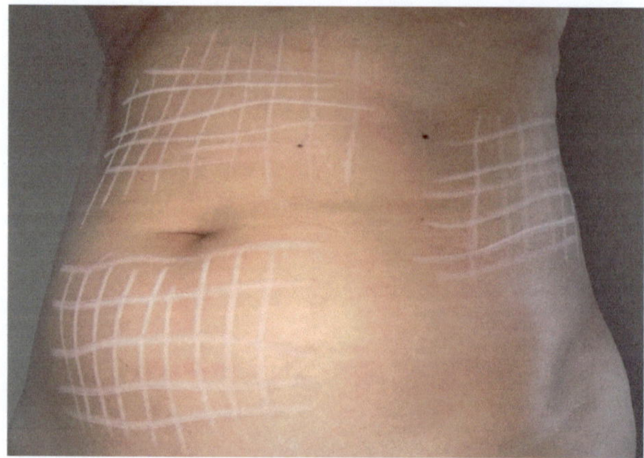

Fig. 26.1 Lines drawn on abdomen showing pattern of mono threads placement

Chapter 27
Procedure for Treatment of Skin on Thighs

1. Cleanse the area to be treated with alcohol or other antiseptic cleanser.
2. Using a white cosmetic pencil and flexible ruler draw lines in a mesh pattern to plan the placement of the threads. Draw the lines according to the length of the threads to be inserted. Plan to use 20 or more threads per side depending on size of area to be treated. Plan to have no more than 1 cm between each thread in order achieve a more uniform improvement. See Fig. 27.1.
3. It is recommended to use Resculpt Medical Threads that are 23 Gauge 60 mm or 90 mm length mono, spring or barbed threads depending on the size and condition of the skin to be treated. Use mono threads if moderately thin skin, spring threads if thin more lax skin needing thickening with collagen, and use barbed threads if desire more fat reduction in thicker skin.
4. Inject local anesthesia subcutaneously in the region to be treated with 2% lidocaine with epinephrine using a cannula after making a pilot hole. Choose the cannula length according to the area that is desired to be treated.
5. Insert the threads along the lines drawn for the pathways of the threads. Be sure to insert in the subcutaneous layer rather than dermal. Do not place too superficially.
6. Even though mono threads or spring threads will be on needles, it is still recommended to create entry holes with an 18 G needle. Puncturing the skin with a 60 mm or 90 mm length thread is difficult even when it is loaded on a sharp end cannula because it is not stiff enough. And of course, if using barbed threads, an entry hole must be made using an 18 Gauge needle since they are usually loaded on blunt cannulas.
7. Once all threads have been placed apply antibiotic ointment to promote faster healing.
8. Prescribe prophylactic antibiotics such as Minocycline 100 mg twice a day for 7 days.

© The Author(s), under exclusive license to Springer Nature Switzerland AG 2023

N. M. Kim, *Non-Surgical Thread Procedures*, https://doi.org/10.1007/978-3-031-36468-6_27

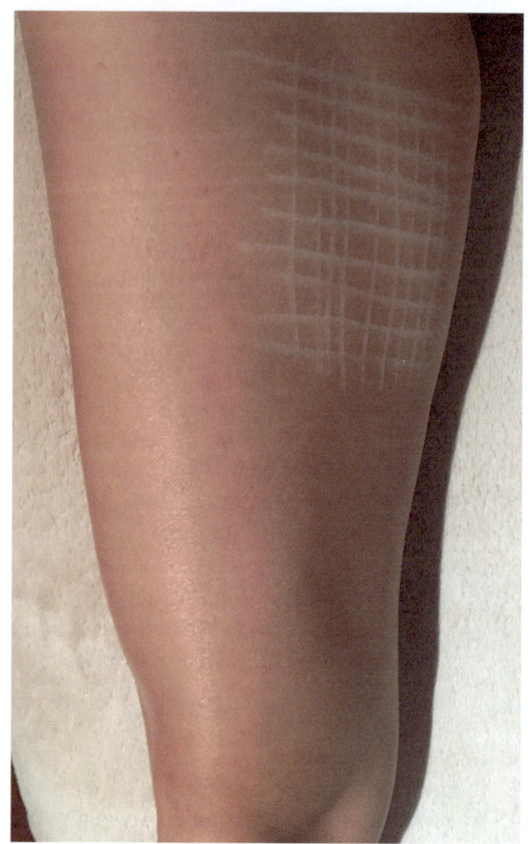

Fig. 27.1 Lines drawn showing pattern of mono thread placement on skin of inner thigh

Chapter 28
Procedure for Treatment of Skin on Knees

1. Cleanse the area on the knees to be treated with alcohol or other antiseptic cleanser.
2. Apply Lidocaine anesthetic cream to the area. Cream with at least 10% or higher lidocaine concentration would be more comfortable for the patient. Allow at least 20 min to become effective.
3. After removing the anesthetic cream, using a white cosmetic pencil, draw lines to indicate where the threads are to be placed. A mesh pattern is best to ensure smooth continuous collagen stimulation. The threads recommended are Resculpt Medical Threads that are 27-gauge 40-mm length blunt cannula threads. Draw the lines of the same length of 40 mm (see Fig. 28.1) Use at least ten threads per area.
4. Figure 28.2 shows a magnified view of the end of the cannula to show that instead of being sharp as is the case for other mono threads, these cannulas have blunt ends. Since these threads are loaded on blunt needles or cannulas which alone cannot puncture the skin, pilot or insertion holes must be made for each thread with a separate needle. Use a needle with a gauge that is slightly larger to make the hole. Since the threads are 27 gauge, use a needle that is 26 gauge to make the holes. Do not puncture too deep and hit the bone. Make the hole just through the skin.
5. Once the pilot or insertion hole is created, insert the thread on the cannula into the subcutaneous tissue through the hole. Repeat for each thread, inserting according to the pattern drawn.
6. Once all the threads are inserted, apply antibiotic ointment to the area.
7. Prescribe prophylactic antibiotics such as Minocycline 100 mg twice a day for 7 days.

© The Author(s), under exclusive license to Springer Nature Switzerland AG 2023

N. M. Kim, *Non-Surgical Thread Procedures*,
https://doi.org/10.1007/978-3-031-36468-6_28

Fig. 28.1 Lines drawn to indicate pattern of thread placement for treating knees skin with mono threads on cannula

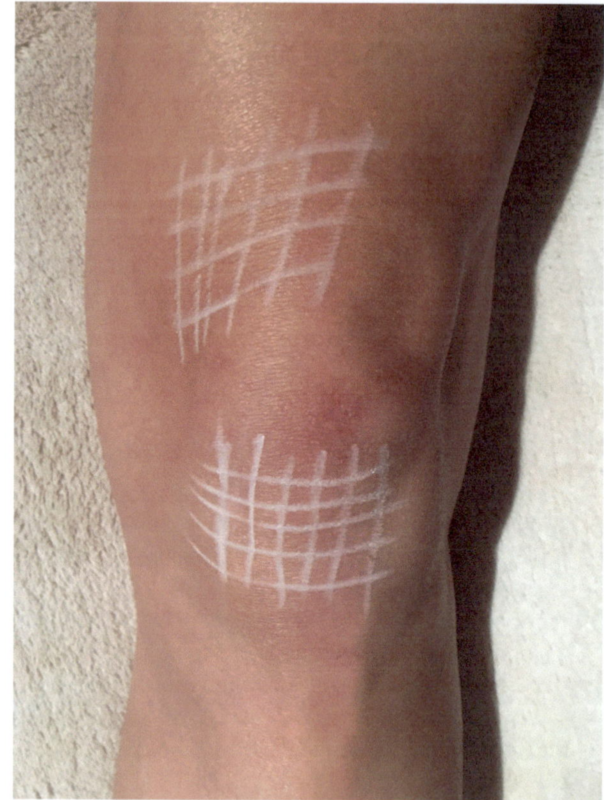

Fig. 28.2 Magnified views of mono threads with blunt end cannula (upper) and sharp end cannula (lower)

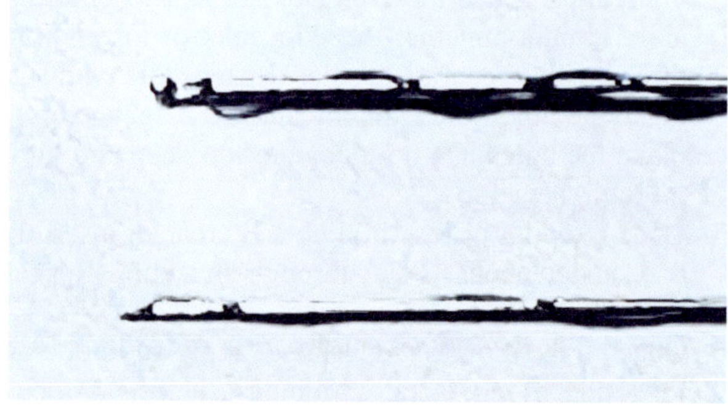

Chapter 29
Procedure for Nose Lift

1. Cleanse nose with alcohol or other antiseptic cleanser.
2. With a white cosmetic pencil, draw a dot where you feel at the tip of the nose, a slight indentation between the alar cartilages. This is the intradomal space at the infratip nodule of the columella. This will be the entry hole site. From this point draw a line of 5 cm length along the bridge towards the radix. See Fig. 29.1.
3. Inject a wheal of anesthetic with 2% Lidocaine with epinephrine using a 30 gauge needle at the tip of the nose where the dot is marked.
4. Using an 18-gauge needle make a pilot hole puncturing through the area of anesthesia.
5. Using a 23-gauge 60-mm cannula enter through the pilot hole to anesthetize the columella down to the base of the nose. Retract and redirect the cannula to anesthetize across the bridge of the nose up the entire length toward the radix.
6. Once anesthesia has been achieved use Resculpt Medical Threads 19-gauge 38-mm nose Profile threads to insert into the columella. Enter through the pilot hole and direct the thread on cannula down towards the base of the nose. Be sure that the thread is completely inserted and pop through the slight resistance at that point of the columellar base and nasolabial junction. It is helpful to pull up with your other hand the columella to create a straight path for the thread to be inserted and for the tip of nose to be stretched forward. Insert up to four threads in this manner into the columella. This will lift the tip of the nose. If the goal is only nose tip lift, then stop here and skip to step 8.
7. For the bridge of the nose use Resculpt Medical Threads 19-gauge 50-mm length nose Profile threads. Enter through the pilot entry hole and direct the cannula with thread facing up along the bridge to the radix. It is helpful to use the other hand to lift the skin slightly while inserting the cannula. Be sure to insert the cannula far enough for the thread to be completely buried under the skin. Repeat with between 6 to 12 threads to build the bridge. Once there is too

© The Author(s), under exclusive license to Springer Nature
Switzerland AG 2023
N. M. Kim, *Non-Surgical Thread Procedures*,
https://doi.org/10.1007/978-3-031-36468-6_29

Fig. 29.1 Dot between alar cartilages representing spot for entry hole. Line drawn on bridge for marking where threads for bridge to be placed

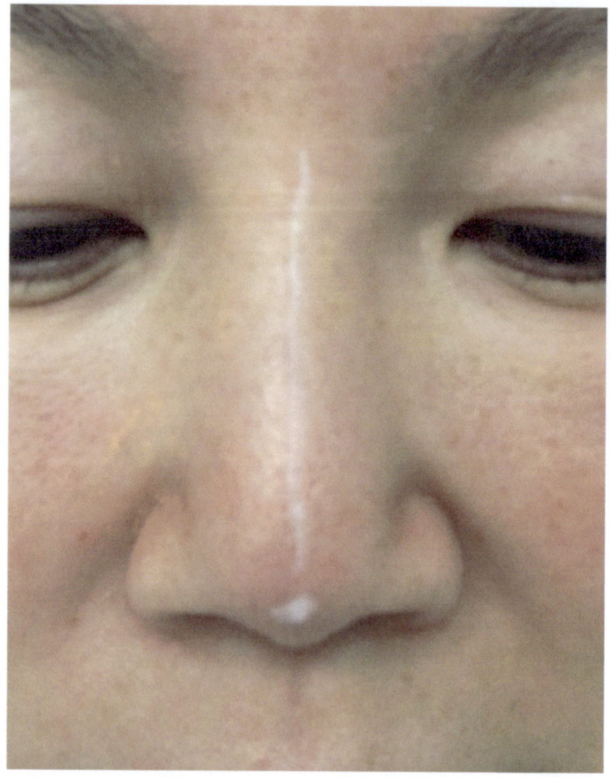

much resistance discontinue adding additional threads. Otherwise, as many as 12 threads can be inserted to give greater height to the bridge.

8. Once all the threads are inserted apply antibiotic ointment to the entry hole. Instruct the patient to avoid touching the nose and to not allow anything to press down on the tip for 1 week and to avoid wearing glasses during that time.

9. Prescribe prophylactic antibiotics such as Minocycline 100 mg twice a day for 5 days.

10. See Figs. 29.2 and 29.3 for before and after photos.

Fig. 29.2 Before and after nose threads for tip and bridge

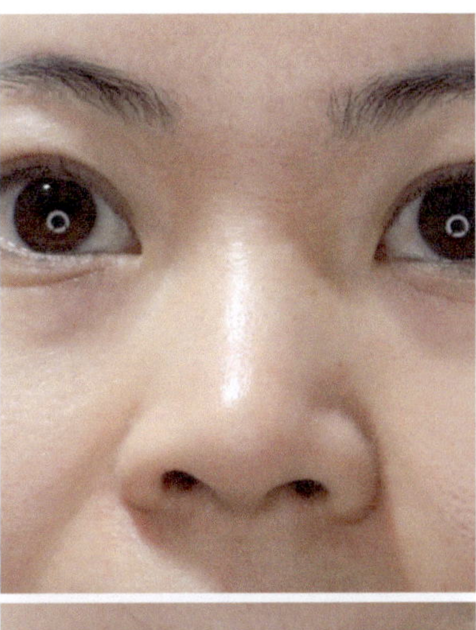

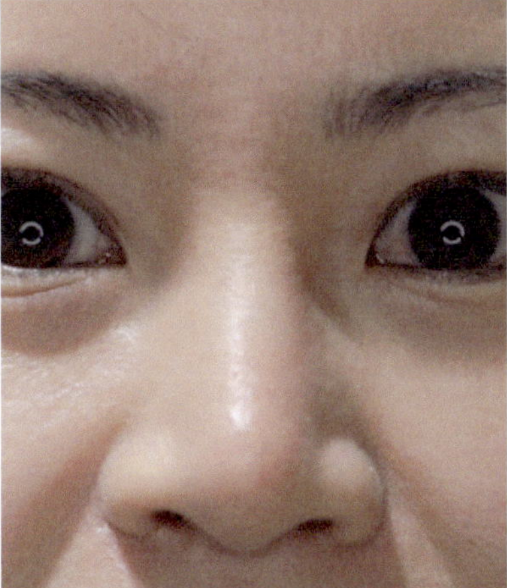

Fig. 29.3 Before and after nose threads for tip and bridge

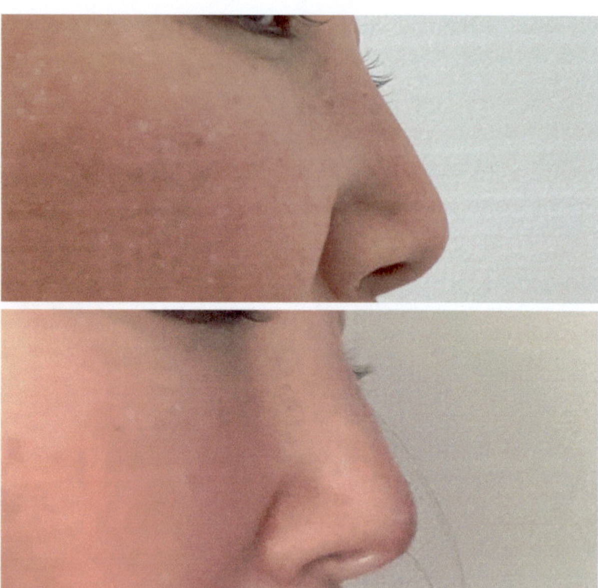

Chapter 30
Patient Consultation and Pre-treatment Counseling

It is important to advise the patient during the consultation which threads would most benefit the patient based on your evaluation. Table 30.1 outlines the basic pretreatment instructions depending on the type of thread to be used. If the patient is a candidate for the barbed threads, it is important to make the patient aware of the post-treatment effects that the patient will feel. For example, describe to the patient where the insertion holes will be. For example, for the cheeks thread lift, the holes will be by the hairline and for the jowls thread lift, behind and below the ear lobe. Inform that these holes will take approximately 5–7 days to heal. They are easily hidden with long hair. There may be some buckling at the site of the insertion holes as well.

Counsel patients regarding the benefits of the procedure. Make certain that the patient's expectations are aligned with the individual potential improvement. For example, many patients will use their one single finger to pull their entire face up and expect that one single thread will lift and create the same effect they are achieving with their single finger pulling. However, this is not how threads work. Be sure that they understand that multiple threads must be utilized to lift each section of the face together. Also explain to them that the threads must pass through the tissue that is to be improved since the collagen stimulation will only occur in those areas of the face where the threads are present. Advise that a significant portion of their improvement in facial contour and skin quality is due to the collagen stimulation by the threads. Explain to them that this is, in fact, the advantage thread lifts have over a surgical facelift. Their face after a thread lift may be more natural appearing and truly undergo anti-aging due to the collagen stimulation.

Advise patients that while they will see some improvement immediately after the procedure, the final results occur 2 months later due to the time needed for the collagen to fully develop and tighten the skin. Patients often ask where the excess skin goes since it is not being cut away as it is in surgery. Explain that the collagen

© The Author(s), under exclusive license to Springer Nature
Switzerland AG 2023

N. M. Kim, *Non-Surgical Thread Procedures*,
https://doi.org/10.1007/978-3-031-36468-6_30

Table 30.1 Pre-procedure instructions for patients based on type of thread to be inserted

Type of threads or area	Pre-treatment instructions and planning
Mono or spiral threads for any area	Avoid alcohol, aspirin, vitamin E, ibuprofen or naproxen, fish oil for 5 days prior
Volumizing or mesh Boost threads for any area	Avoid alcohol, aspirin, vitamin E, ibuprofen or naproxen, fish oil for 5 days prior
Barbed threads for face or neck	Avoid alcohol, aspirin, vitamin E, ibuprofen or naproxen, fish oil for 5 days prior
	Do not plan any dental procedure for 2 weeks afterwards
	Do not plan for any facial procedure for 1 week afterwards
	Do not plan for any massage procedure for where face is placed inside circular pillow
	Recommend to not schedule procedure if any significant social events during the following 1 week

stimulation helps to shrink the excess skin. In addition, the excess lax skin is redistributed towards the periphery of the face more evenly rather than accumulated in the jowls or nasolabial folds in the front of the face. Be sure to explain to patients that also once the procedure is done the improvement in terms of lift immediately after the procedure will be more than what they will see once the swelling goes down 1–2 weeks later. However, 1–2 months later after the collagen stimulation occurs, the lift will then be increased again due to contraction of the skin from collagen increase.

When doing consultations for neck lift with barbed threads, it is important to give realistic expectations to patients who have significant bulk or very large double chin. The neck is a challenging area when it is significantly heavy. Improvement may be limited to 30–50% depending on how bulky the neck tissue is. This is unlike the face, which almost always has very satisfactory improvement. Facial fat does not vary between one person to the next as much as the size of a neck. Therefore, in patients who are very heavy in their neck area it is important to align their expectations with the possible outcome. Ideal patients are those who have laxity of skin but only mild to moderate amount of fat.

For patients who are interested in the barbed thread lift for cheeks, jowls, neck or eyebrows, it is important to give some information regarding what to expect after the procedure in order for patients to schedule the procedure at an appropriate time for them. Although after the barbed thread lift, there is usually not significant bruising, there is a possibility of swelling and discomfort that may preclude them from important social activities. Since it is necessary to protect the threads from being broken or loosened, it is important to have the patient schedule the procedure at a time that will allow rest and recovery that will provide optimal results from the treatment.

30.1 Specific Instructions Regarding Barbed Threads for Cheeks, Jowls and Neck

Inform patients that their face or neck will feel tight for 1–2 weeks after the procedure. There will be discomfort with chewing and facial expressions as well as neck rotation. Advise patients to avoid eating foods that require significant chewing such as beef, chicken, and bread. Ask patients to limit diet to soft foods such as fish, well cooked vegetables, soup, and other soft foods. Inform patients that they should not have any dental procedures scheduled for 2 weeks after the procedure. Facial massages or any other massage that requires the face to be put in a pillow must be avoided for 1–2 weeks after the procedure. The first 24 h will be the most uncomfortable where even flossing or brushing teeth may be uncomfortable. Advise the patient to rest during the remainder of the day after the procedure. There is no significant bruising and even swelling may be tolerable, however, there may be discomfort that will preclude socializing during the first day. In addition, patients should be advised not to schedule the procedure prior to any events that will require them to have vigorous exercise that will cause them to strain their face or rotate their head to a significant degree. Vigorous exercise should be avoided for 1–2 weeks. Mild exercise such as on an elliptical machine or walking is allowed and not harmful, however, vigorous sports or yoga is not advised. These instructions are for the purposes of ensuring that the threads do no become broken and that the patient experiences less discomfort.

30.2 Specific Instructions Regarding Barbed Threads for Eyebrows

Because the threads will pass through the tissues of the forehead to lift the eyebrows, it is important for patients to be aware that there may be a significant amount of swelling after the procedure that is easily visible due to the fact that the forehead has very little fat to hide swelling. The swelling is visible against the bone more so than in other parts of the face. It is important for patients therefore to schedule the treatment when they will not feel self-conscious about this swelling. The swelling will last for approximately 1–2 weeks and consists of irregular contours on the forehead. Therefore, it is advisable that patients do not schedule the procedure immediately prior to any important social events. It is also recommended that patients have had botulinum toxin or receive treatment in order to immobilize the forehead muscles. Doing so will allow the threads to maintain their hold with less risk of breakage or loosening of thread position. This will also make it more comfortable for the patient as well since they will be not creating more tension with expression.

30.3   Instructions Regarding Body Threads

For patients receiving threads in body areas, it is important to inform patients that there is discomfort after the procedure particularly because it is very hard to limit movement. Daily tasks can cause discomfort. It is important to limit the amount of exercise particularly during the first 2 weeks. Patients must consider this in terms of scheduling their procedure at a time when they can avoid vigorous activity after the procedure. Patients should also be informed that there is more risk of hyperpigmentation at the insertion sites and body areas than in the face, particularly with ethnicities such as Asian, Hispanic, Middle Eastern, and African American.

Chapter 31
Post-procedure Instructions for Patients

(a) If patient received barbed threads for eyebrows: All instructions are for 1 week unless otherwise stated (see Table 31.1).

- Avoid rubbing vigorously in the area of the forehead and hairline when washing face or washing hair.
- Avoid wearing tight fitting hats or caps and avoid sleeping on sides of face.
- Avoid allowing animation of forehead muscles. It is recommended to use botulinum toxin to decrease muscle activity in the forehead.
- Apply antibiotic ointment to the insertion holes daily until healed, usually 5–7 days.
- If using ice to relieve discomfort apply ice gently without using significant pressure on the threads.
- Tylenol is best if opt to take medicine for discomfort. Avoid medications that can cause thinning of the blood such as ibuprofen, naproxen, aspirin.

(b) If received barbed threads for cheeks and jowls: All instructions are for 1 week unless otherwise stated.

- Avoid massaging the face when washing. Avoid using exfoliating scrubs for 1 week.
- Avoid vigorous activity that causes strong animation of facial muscles.
- Avoid eating foods that require significant chewing such as beef, chicken, bread, crunchy foods. Fish, noodles, rice, soup, and other soft foods is best.
- Avoid sleeping on sides of face. Try to sleep on back.
- Avoid dental procedures for 2 weeks afterwards.
- Avoid getting massages that require you to be face down on a massage table.
- Avoid water sports activities until the insertion sites are healed. Avoid excess sun as well to prevent hyperpigmentation of the insertion sites.
- If using ice to relieve discomfort, apply ice gently without using significant pressure on the threads.

© The Author(s), under exclusive license to Springer Nature Switzerland AG 2023

N. M. Kim, *Non-Surgical Thread Procedures*,
https://doi.org/10.1007/978-3-031-36468-6_31

Table 31.1 Post procedure instructions for patients

Type of threads or area treated	Post-care instructions for patients
Mono or spiral threads	Keep clean but may use concealer if desired.
Mesh threads	Apply antibiotic ointment to insertion holes daily.
Barbed threads eyebrows	Apply antibiotic ointment to insertion holes daily.
	Avoid vigorous massage when washing face or hairline in area of threads for 1 week. Avoid excessive expressive movements of eyebrows for 1 week.
	Take antibiotics as prescribed for 1 week.
Barbed threads cheeks, jowls, and/or neck	Avoid foods that require significant chewing such as beef, chicken, bread and crunchy vegetables. Maintain a soft food diet for 1 week after procedure.
	Avoid sleeping on sides of face for 1 week after procedure.
	Avoid dental or other facial procedure for 2 weeks after procedure.
	Avoid exercise that may cause significant movements of head and neck.
	Take antibiotics as prescribed for 1 week.

- Apply antibiotic ointment to the insertion holes daily until healed, usually for 5–7 days.
- Tylenol is best if opting to take medicine for discomfort. Avoid medications that can cause thinning of the blood such as ibuprofen, naproxen, aspirin.

(c) If received barbed threads on neck: All instructions are for 1 week unless otherwise stated (see Table 31.1).

- Avoid vigorous sports activities that require significant rotation of the head. Mild activity that allows you to keep head still such as riding a stationary bicycle or elliptical machine is best.
- Avoid sleeping on sides of face, try to sleep on back.
- Avoid eating foods that require significant chewing such as beef, chicken, bread, and crunchy foods. Fish, noodles, rice, soup, and other soft foods is best.
- Avoid dental procedures for 2 weeks afterwards.
- Avoid getting massages that require you to be face down on a massage table.
- Avoid water sports activities until the insertion sites are healed.
- Avoid excess sun to prevent hyperpigmentation of the insertion sites.
- Apply antibiotic ointment to the insertion holes daily until healed, usually 5–7 days.
- If using ice to relieve discomfort apply ice gently without using significant pressure on the threads.
- Tylenol is best if opting to take medicine for discomfort. Avoid medications that can cause thinning of the blood such as ibuprofen, naproxen, aspirin.

(d) If received barbed treads for body areas: All instructions are for 1 week unless otherwise stated (See Table 31.1).

- Avoid vigorous activities with the body part that was treated. It is important to limit amount of tension on threads until pain and discomfort is decreased which usually takes 1–2 weeks.
- Avoid significant pressure on the area as much as possible. For example, if butt lift is done try to decrease the amount of sitting on hard surfaces.
- Avoid water sports activities until the insertion sites are healed.
- Avoid excess sun to prevent hyperpigmentation of the insertion sites.
- Apply antibiotic ointment to the insertion holes daily until healed, usually 5–7 days.
- If using ice to relieve discomfort apply ice gently without applying significant pressure on the threads.
- Tylenol is best if opting to take medicine for discomfort. Avoid medications that can cause thinning of the blood such as ibuprofen, naproxen, Aspirin.

(e) If received mono threads and/or mesh threads (see Table 31.1):

- Apply antibiotic ointment to the insertion holes or area daily until healed, usually 5–7 days.
- If using ice to relieve discomfort, apply ice gently without using significant pressure on the threads. Avoid sleeping on sides of face.
- Tylenol is best if opting to take medicine for discomfort. Avoid medications that can cause thinning of the blood such as ibuprofen, naproxen, aspirin.
- With these threads it is not necessary to limit activities except only for personal preference and discomfort level. There is no risk to harming the threads or the result by engaging in physical activity.
- Avoid water sports activities until the insertion sites are healed.
- Avoid excess sun to prevent hyperpigmentation of the insertion sites.

Chapter 32
Complications and Their Management

32.1 Dimpling

Mild dimpling in the skin may be unavoidable in some patients. When the barbed threads are holding the tissue in one area and pulling together a significant amount of tissue from another area, the dimpling can occur and be noticeable initially. However, usually 1–2 weeks after the procedure, the dimpling disappears as the swollen tissue recedes and tissue contraction occurs. See Fig. 32.1 for example of mild dimpling. Significant dimpling that is deeper or over an extended length of tissue of greater than 2 cm should be manually released to avoid prolonged discomfort and dissatisfaction with appearance. Manual release can be achieved by massaging the skin along the thread pathway in the direction away from the insertion site with moderate pressure (see Video 33.3 in Chap. 33). More pressure can be used as needed until release is felt and seen. Sometimes, the release is easier to achieve once the end of the thread has been cut as well. Dimpling sometimes is not noticed until days or even a few weeks after the procedure and swelling has subsided. It is still possible to release the dimpling in these instances with use of enough pressure. Some lubrication of skin with aloe vera or alcohol gel can make is easier and more comfortable for the patient when the manuever is performed for release.

32.2 Infection

It is rare to see infection with thread procedures. Most commonly if there is an infection, it is limited to the insertion site where possibly an ingrown hair has triggered it, or if the thread end did not get buried under the skin, causing the insertion hole to be unable to heal and close. If a finger is placed over the insertion hole site, a sharp point of the thread can be felt even if not seen, indicating that the

© The Author(s), under exclusive license to Springer Nature
Switzerland AG 2023
N. M. Kim, *Non-Surgical Thread Procedures*,
https://doi.org/10.1007/978-3-031-36468-6_32

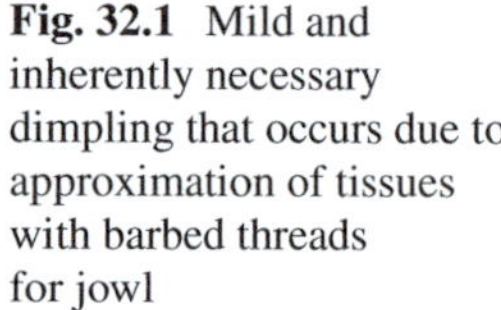

Fig. 32.1 Mild and inherently necessary dimpling that occurs due to approximation of tissues with barbed threads for jowl

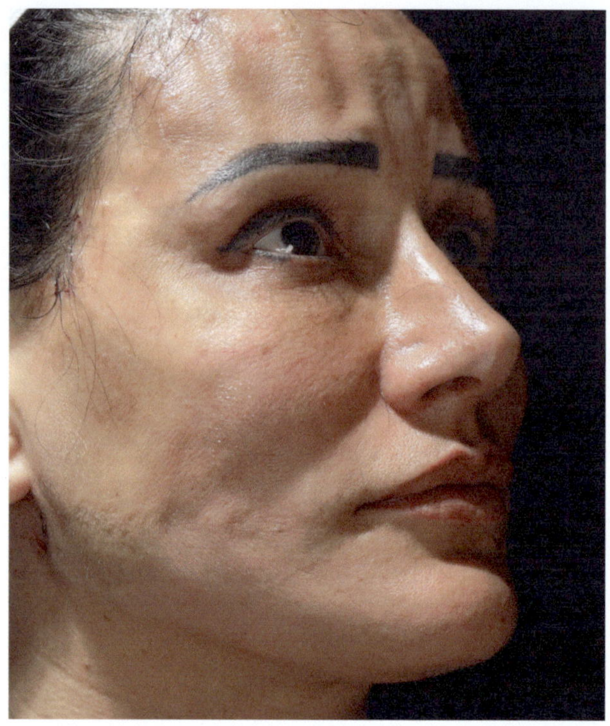

thread end did not bury under the skin. Patients may report redness, swelling and tenderness in the area or spreading from it. They may report drainage from the site. The infection can occur even weeks after the procedure if it is due to ingrown hair for which there is more risk in patients with curly hair. Usually, fever is not reported, and the infection is slowly progressing. Generally, the thread does not need to be removed. Treating with a course of antibiotics such as doxycycline or minocycline is usually adequate. If the thread end is protruding, then it of course needs to be cut so that it will bury under the skin and allow the hole to heal. Cutting the end of the thread and a course of antibiotics rather than removing the thread will often successfully resolve the infection.

The recommended antibiotics include doxycycline or minocycline. Clindamycin or Amoxicillin may also be used. A 7–10-day course is recommended. It is important to make sure the patient is not allergic to the medication. It is important to reassure the patient as significant anxiety can be generated surrounding any issues with the face and post-procedure complications.

32.3   Thread End Protruding Out of Skin

It is possible for the end of the thread to have not buried under the skin and remain protruding slightly out of the insertion hole preventing the hole from healing. In this case it is also possible for mild infection to occur due to the thread end being a nidus of infection. Sometimes if the thread end still has some barbs on it, it may even catch onto something and be pulled out even more, causing puckering of the skin. When placing a finger over the insertion hole site one may feel a sharp material which is the end of the thread. See Fig. 32.2, for example, of thread end protruding out through skin noticed more than 1 week after the procedure. If this is the case that thread must be cut closer to the skin, so that the thread end can bury itself under the skin. Forceps must be used to grasp the end of the thread and pulled while the scissors are placed down with pressure downward onto the skin to cut the thread as low as possible. This should allow the thread to bury itself. Figure 32.3 shows the end of the thread cut off. If there was an infection present, then an antibiotic course

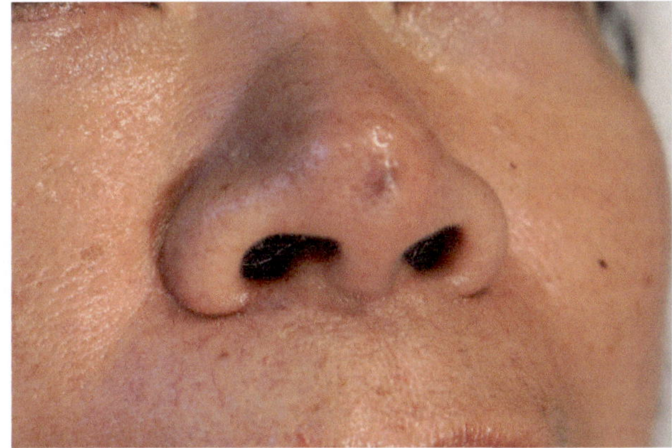

Fig. 32.2 Appearance of skin when thread end protruding through hole and not allowing hole to heal more than 1 week after the procedure. This requires the thread end to be cut closer to skin to bury the end so that skin can close over it

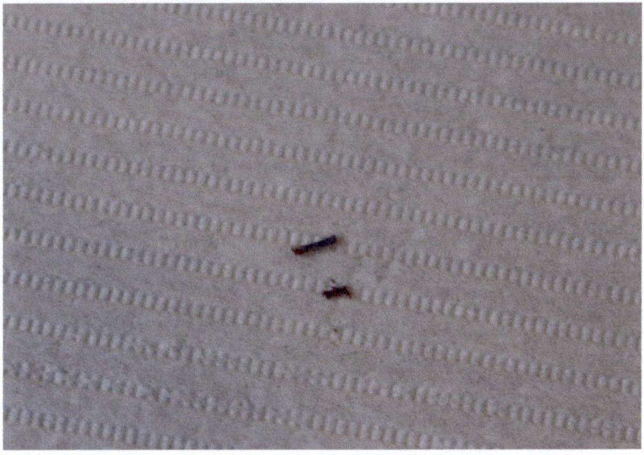

Fig. 32.3 The end of thread that was protruding through the skin in Fig. 32.2 after it is cut off

of Minocycline 100 mg twice a day for 7 days should be sufficient to clear the infection and allow healing of the hole. The entire thread does not necessarily need to be removed unless there is no improvement after antibiotics.

32.4   Thread Breakage

It is possible within the first few weeks after the procedure for the thread to break. This may occur if the patient is not careful and compliant with instructions to be gentle with the area and avoid activities that can cause loosening or breakage of the threads. It may become apparent that a thread broke when a sudden change in the tightness of the skin or an abnormal appearance of the skin is noticed. The patient may report feeling a click or some other sensation such as a snap. It may also become apparent immediately after or later that the free end of the thread has migrated and become more superficial. When this happens, the thread may become visible through the skin as well (see Fig. 32.4). If the thread is not visible, then it does not need to be removed. However, a new thread to tighten the skin in the area may be warranted. If the thread end does migrate and or become visible through the

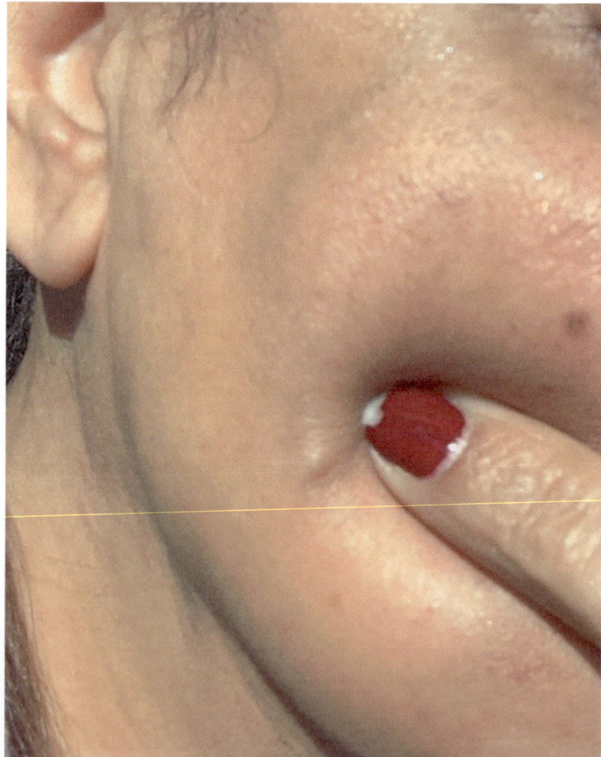

Fig. 32.4 Thread visible through skin due to breakage and migration more superficially

skin, then that thread end must be removed. To remove the thread that is visible make a wheal at or near the visible end of the thread. Using an 18-gauge needle make a hole at the site of anesthesia. It may be necessary to puncture multiple times in the same location to create a slightly larger hole so that the thread may extrude out. Attempt to massage and push the thread out through the hole. It is helpful to try to stretch the skin over the protruding thread and manipulate the thread to make it migrate out through the hole created. You may also use a vein hook as shown in Fig. 32.5 to pull the end of the thread out through the hole. This may take some time and patience. Once a piece of the end is palpable or visible through the hole, use forceps to grasp it and pull it out. It is often very easy to pull out as it is often free and no longer attached with barbs to the tissue. Figure 32.6 shows the broken end of a thread that was removed from the site shown in Fig. 32.4. Apply antibiotic ointment to the hole.

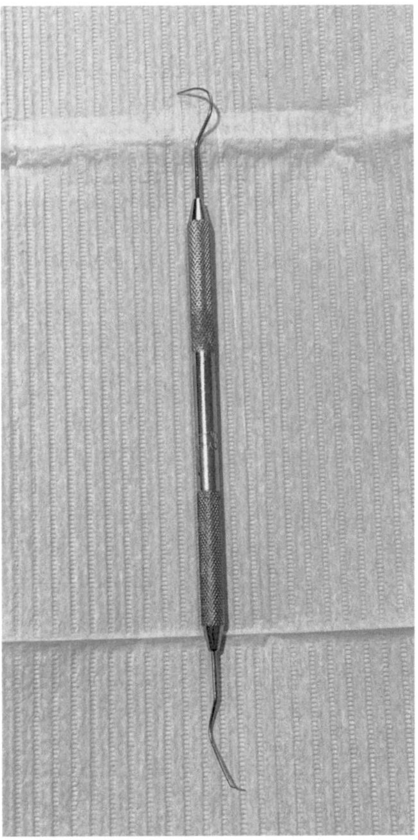

Fig. 32.5 Vein hook that can be used to pull on thread and encourage end of thread to come out through hole in order to remove it

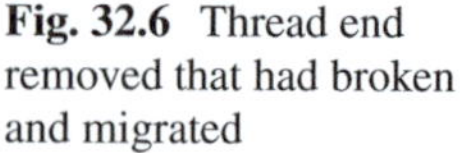

Fig. 32.6 Thread end removed that had broken and migrated

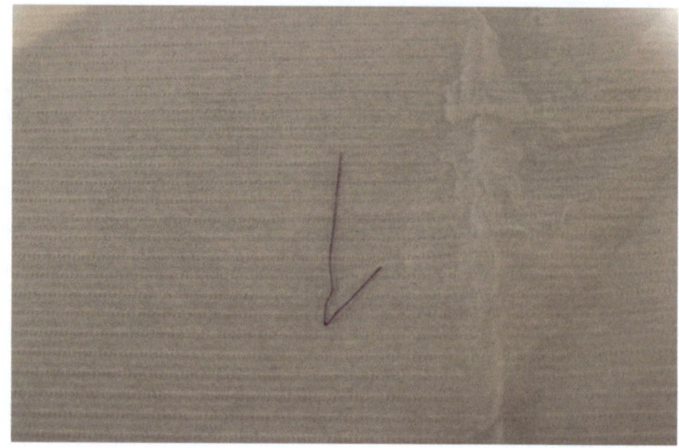

32.5   Thread Visible Through Skin

If the thread is visible through the skin after barbed thread procedure this may be due to too superficial of a placement or thread migration due to breakage. If after mesh thread insertion, the thread end seems to tent up the skin, this may be due to the thread not being placed far enough inside away from the insertion hole or due to allowing the thread end to be still initially outside of the hole but then bury itself under the skin with too close placement near the hole. In such cases it is preferable for the patient to have the thread removed. The thread end is usually visible and palpable through the skin with manipulation of the skin. Inject anesthesia at the site where the thread end is palpable as close to it as possible. Then while manipulating the skin or pinching the skin to make the thread end more visible, puncture the skin with an 18 g needle as close as possible to the end of the thread as if to create a tract where the thread can pass through. It may be necessary to puncture several times to make the hole slightly larger to make it easier for the thread to pass through. Once the hole is created, manipulate or massage the skin to encourage the thread to pass through the hole. It is possible to use a vein hook as shown in Fig. 32.5 to pull some thread so that the end comes out of the hole. All that is needed is for the end of thread to slightly protrude through the hole so that you can grasp it with forceps and pull it out. It is important to use your fingers and be sensitive to feeling for the sharpness of the end in order to be aware of when the thread end has popped out. Please see Fig. 32.7 showing thread visible and site to make hole.

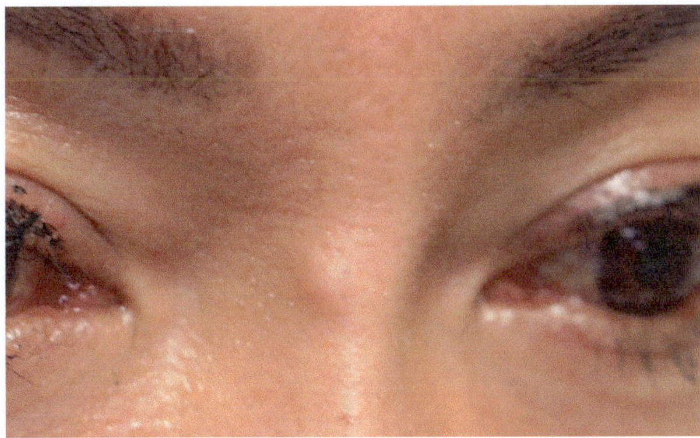

Fig. 32.7 Thread end visibly tenting up the skin from beneath

32.6 Thread Migration

If a thread has broken, often the free end or distal end of the thread relative to the entry site will migrate since it is no longer connected to the rest of the thread that is anchored. The free end can migrate quite a distance even to another area of the face altogether. For example, a portion of thread that broke away from a thread that was in the jowl region can migrate down below the chin. When this occurs, if the thread is visible enough that it is bothersome to the patient, it is best to remove it. The technique described in the previous section on how to remove a thread visible through the skin can be used to remove the migrated portion of the thread. If the thread is not significantly visible or bothersome to the patient, the thread can be allowed to remain, and will over time become less visible as it becomes absorbed. This may take several months. However, if the patient does not mind or it is in a location where not visible, this may be an acceptable option.

32.7 Excess Buckling

In some cases where there is much laxity of the skin, and in an attempt to approximate the lax skin tightly to the anchoring site, significant buckling or bunching of skin may occur. In other words, a large amount of skin is accumulated at the anchoring site (see Fig. 32.8). This may be a necessary process in these cases, in order to gain a satisfactory result in terms of tightening the lax skin of the jowls or neck. Some degree of buckling is desirable to achieve this satisfactory result. And in most cases, the buckling will resolve in 1–2 weeks' time as the threads soften, the swelling resolves and the tissue contracts. Even in the patient shown in Fig. 32.8, the buckling resolved after only 1 week and appeared socially acceptable already after only

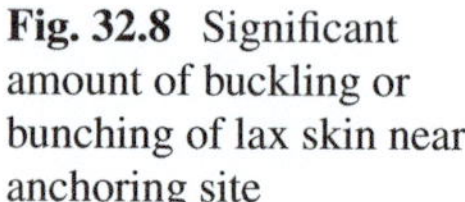

Fig. 32.8 Significant amount of buckling or bunching of lax skin near anchoring site

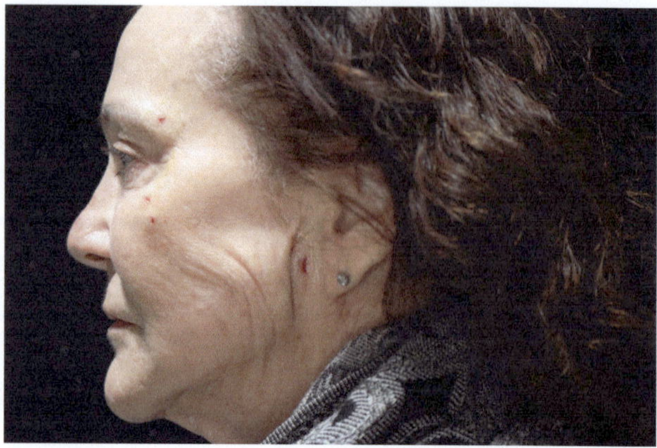

a few days. However, in some cases there may be too much buckling that does not resolve enough and causes residual discomfort to the patient. In these cases, it is still possible to manually release some of the tension if less than 3 weeks since the procedure. Placing a significant amount of pressure on the buckled region with a massaging motion away from the insertion site, will often release partially some of the barbs from their hold enough to reduce some of the buckling. Any remaining buckling will surely resolve over time even if it may take several months to do so. Reassurance to the patient will be paramount in such cases.

Chapter 33
Case Examples

33.1 Patient #1

This patient has thick skin but early signs of cheek, jowl, and eyelid laxity, fat loss with deep nasolabial folds, undereye hollowing, and neck laxity. She also desired her nose bridge to be more projected forward. Figures 33.1, 33.2, 33.3, 33.4, and 33.5 show her before procedure photos.

Figure 33.6 shows the lines drawn indicating the planned areas for thread insertion. She received these threads as listed below.

- 20 G × 60 mm × 8 barbed threads for eyebrow lift (not shown here but was performed)
- For nose lift: 19 G × 38 mm × 4 nose threads for columella and 20 G × 50 mm × 12 nose threads for nose bridge
- 19 G × 38 mm × 4 mesh threads for undereye
- 19 G × 38 mm × 4 mesh threads for nasolabial folds
- 18 G × 100 mm × 4 barbed threads for cheeks
- 18 G × 100 mm × 4 barbed threads for jowls
- 18 G × 100 mm × 4 for neck submental region

Figures 33.7, 33.8, 33.9, 33.10, and 33.11 show photos of patient immediately after the thread procedures. Note the buckling and mild dimpling that can occur with a properly done procedure.

Supplementary Information The online version contains supplementary material available at https://doi.org/10.1007/978-3-031-36468-6_33.

© The Author(s), under exclusive license to Springer Nature Switzerland AG 2023
N. M. Kim, *Non-Surgical Thread Procedures*,
https://doi.org/10.1007/978-3-031-36468-6_33

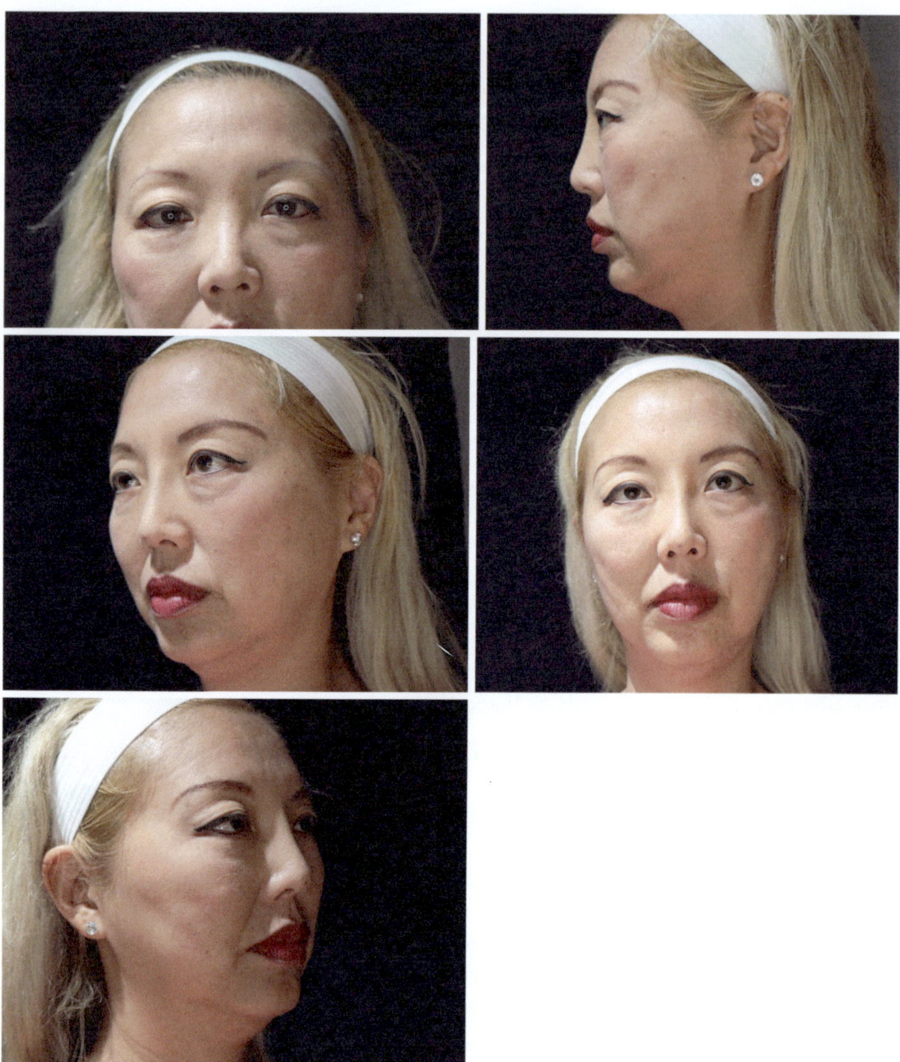

Figs. 33.1–33.5 Patient #1 photos of face and neck prior to her thread lift procedures

Figures 33.12, 33.13, 33.14, 33.15, and 33.16 show photos of the same patient, 1 month after the procedure. These demonstrate that the buckling and dimpling resolve. Improvement in laxity and change in nose contour is already seen at 1 month.

Figures 33.17, 33.18, 33.19, 33.20, and 33.21 show photos of Patient #1 at 6 months after the procedure. Note the continued improvement in laxity and overall shrinkage of the size of the lower face.

Fig. 33.6 Patient #1 with lines drawn indicating the planned areas for threads insertions

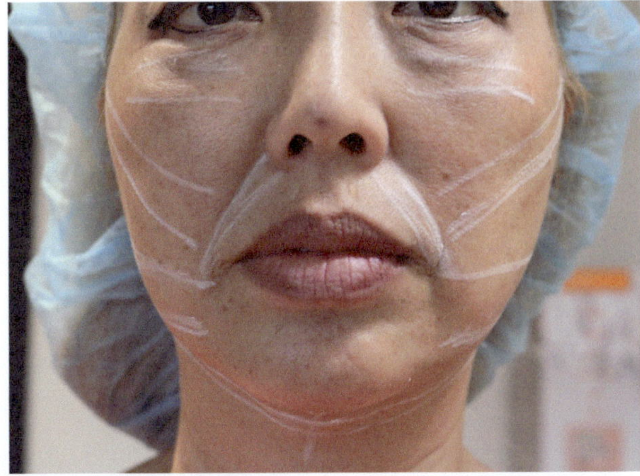

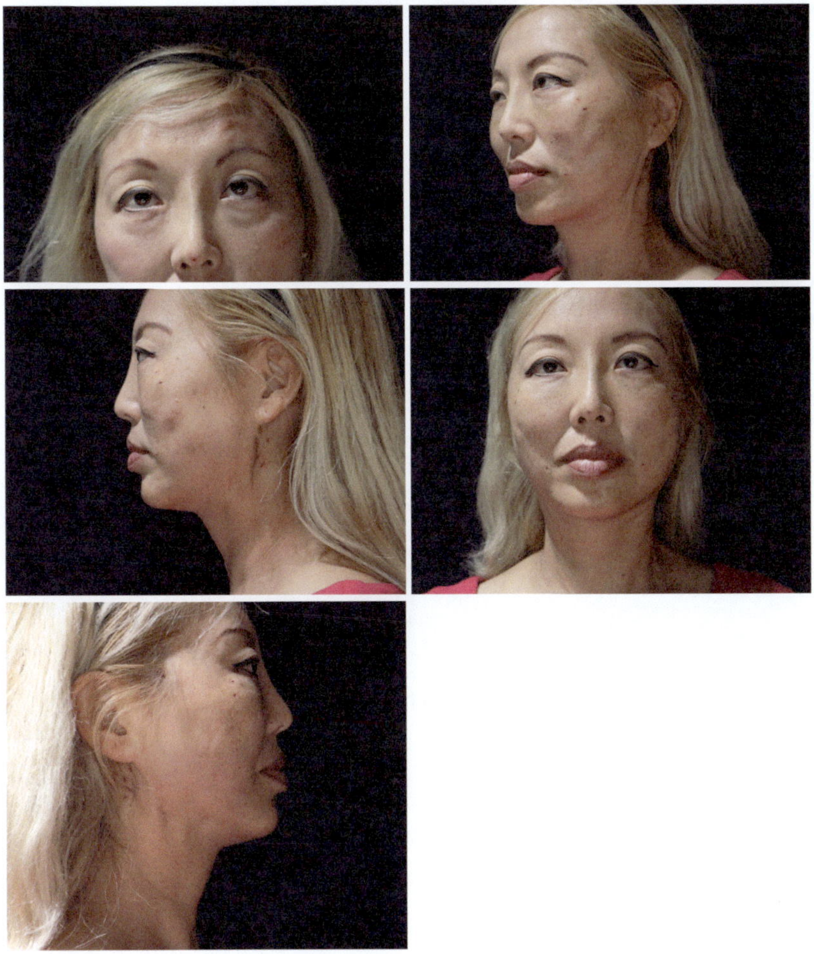

Figs. 33.7–33.11 Patient #1 immediately after thread lift procedures

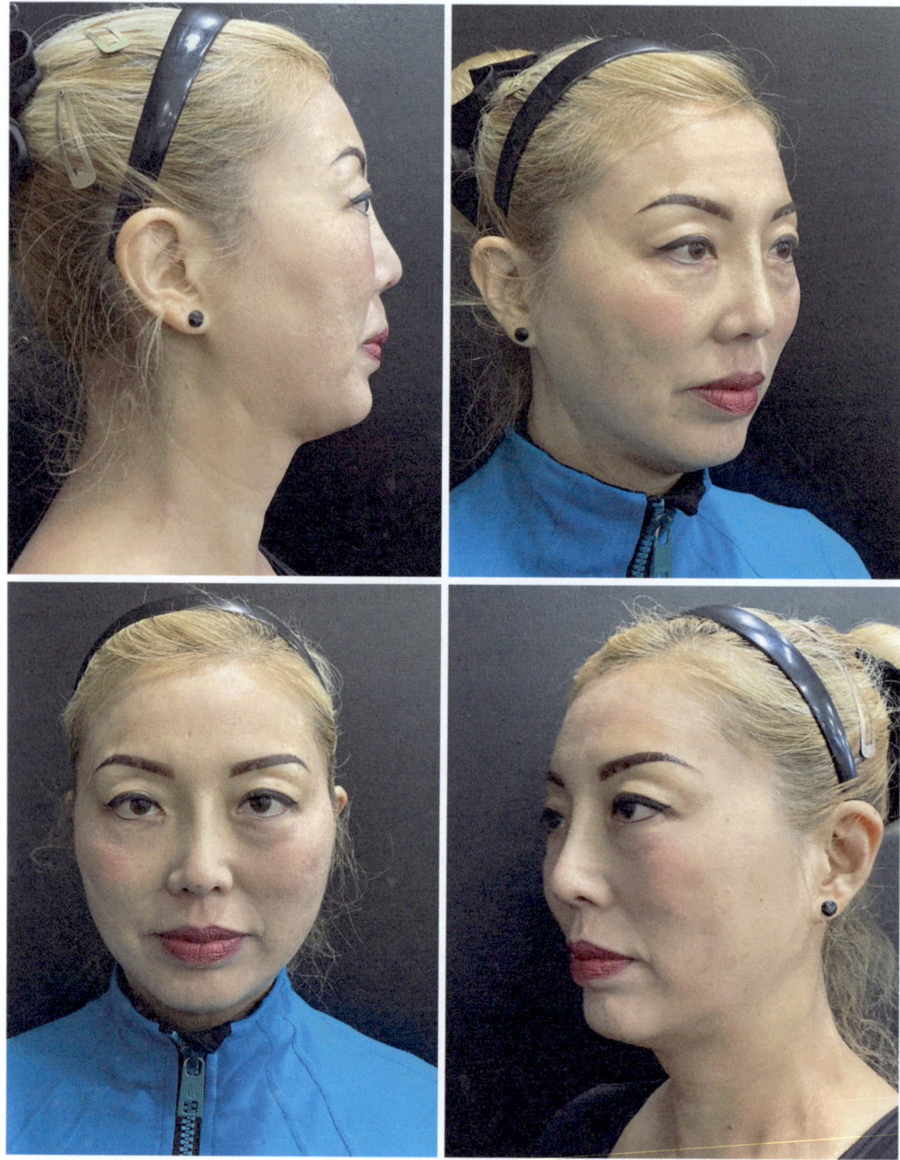

Figs. 33.12–33.16 Patient #1 1 month after the thread lift procedures

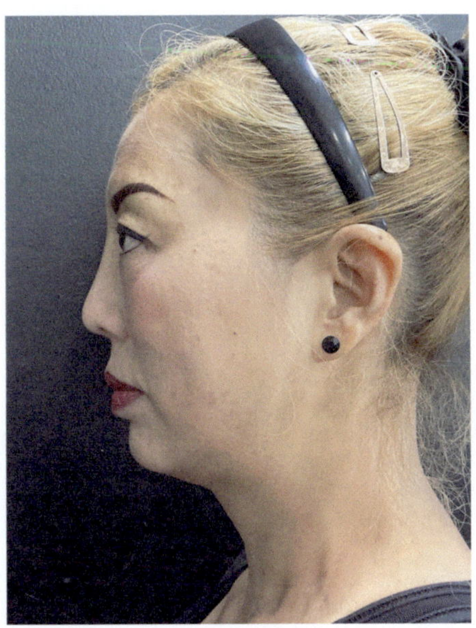

Figs. 33.12–33.16 (continued)

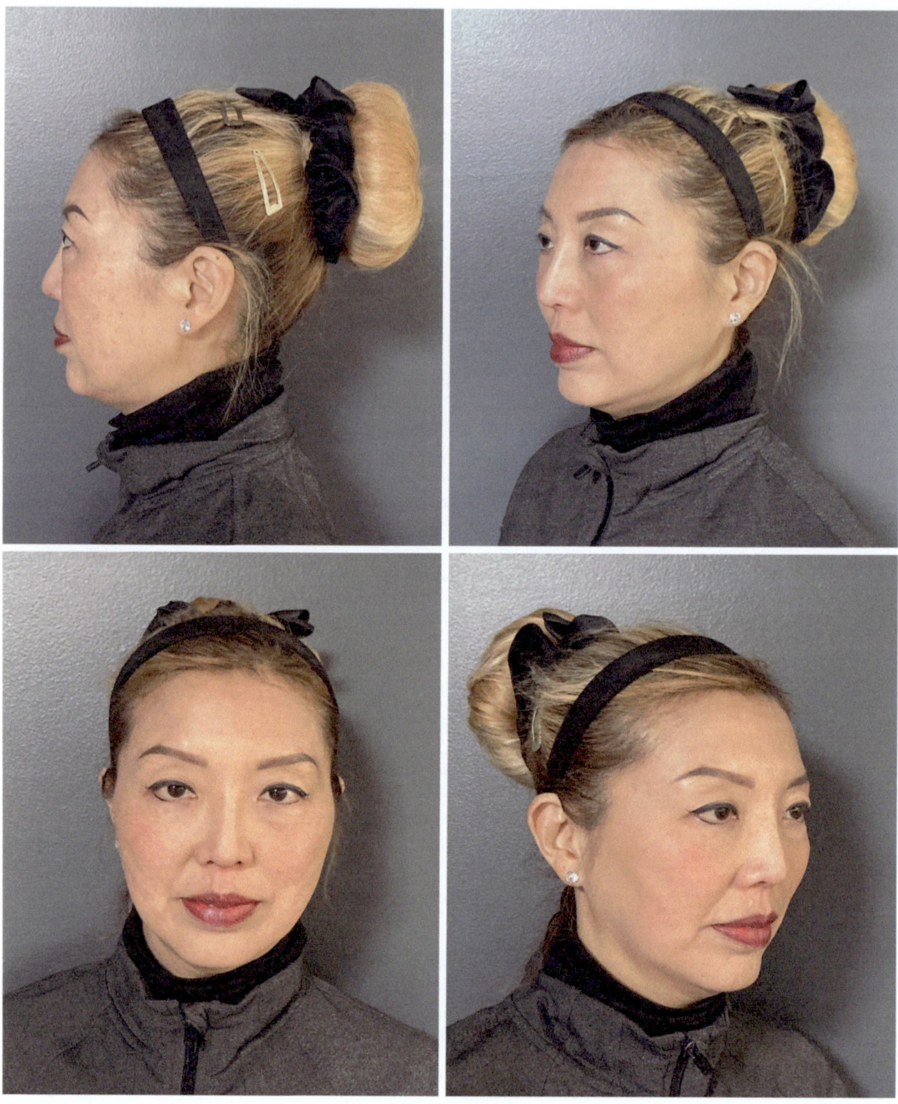

Figs. 33.17–33.21 Patient #1 at 6 months after the thread lift procedures

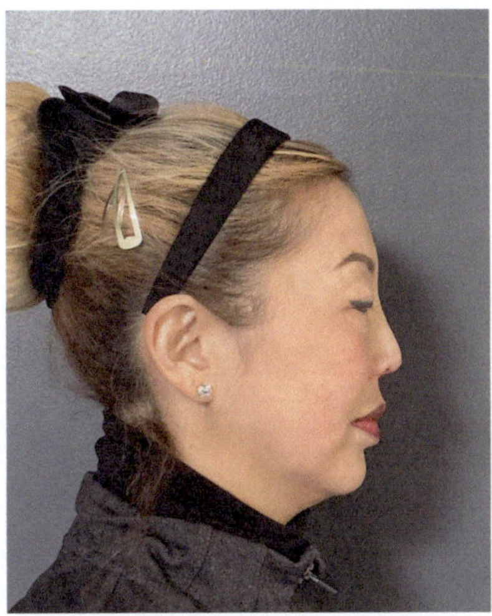

Figs. 33.17–33.21 (continued)

33.2 Patient #2

This patient has skin with more laxity than patient #1. She received treatment with barbed threads for her cheeks and jowls laxity similarly as patient #1. However, to address the laxity of her skin in the jowls, a double layered treatment with thicker gauge threads in the deeper subcutaneous layer and thinner gauge in the upper subcutaneous later was performed. A double layered treatment is very helpful when there are pouches or pockets of lax skin and fat that the patients desire to have minimized.

Figures 33.22, 33.23, 33.24, 33.25, and 33.26 show the patient's face prior to the procedure.

The patient received the following threads:

- 21 G × 90 mm × 4 barbed threads for cheeks
- 21 G × 90 mm × 6 barbed threads for upper layer jowls
- 20 G × 100 mm × 1 barbed thread with D type cannula to precisely target upper layer fatty pouch on right jowl.
- 18 G × 100 mm × 4 barbed thread for deeper layer jowls

Figures 33.27, 33.28, 33.29, 33.30, and 33.31 show the patient's face immediately after the procedure. Note mild dimpling and buckling which may be worrisome to the patient. However, the patient must be reassured that this is temporary and necessary to gain optimal results. The buckling and dimpling will resolve significantly within 1 week.

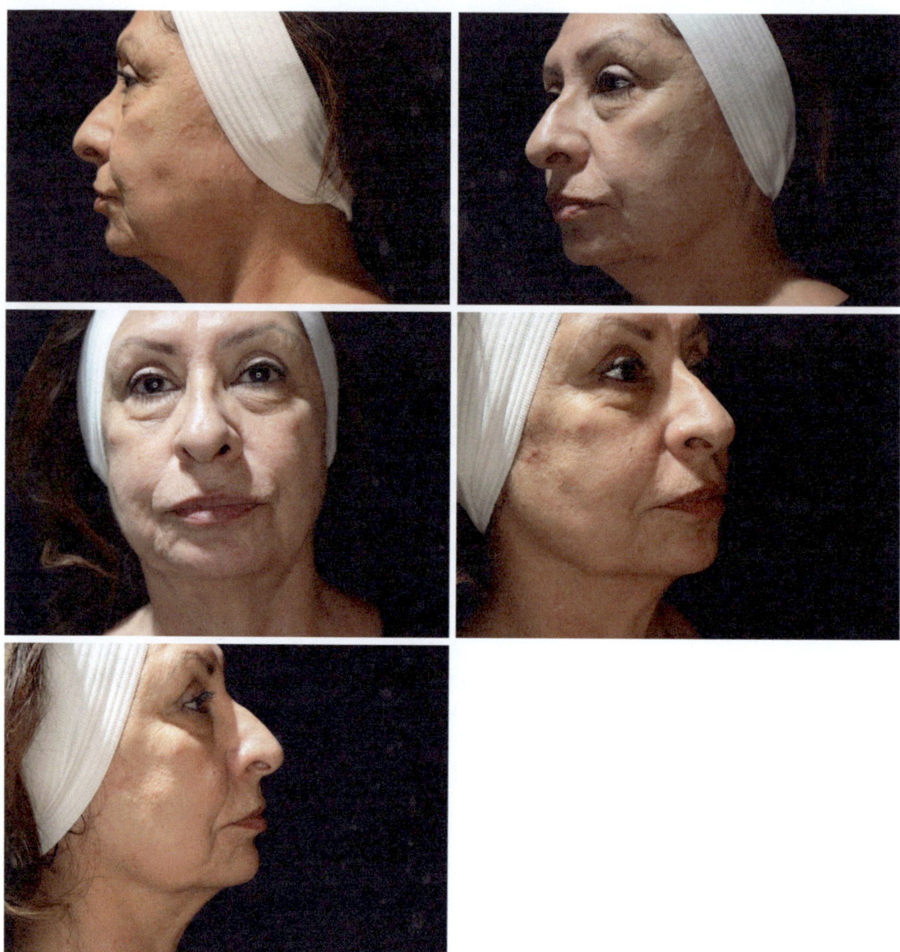

Figs. 33.22–33.26 Patient #2 immediately prior to thread lift procedures

Notice the significant resolution of dimpling and buckling seen after 2 weeks, as shown in Figs. 33.32, 33.33, 33.34, 33.35, and 33.36. Improvement in face shape and contour can also be seen already at 2 weeks.

At 1 month after the procedure, even more significant smoothing of face contours and decrease in laxity can be seen, as shown in Figs. 33.37, 33.38, 33.39, 33.40 and 33.41.

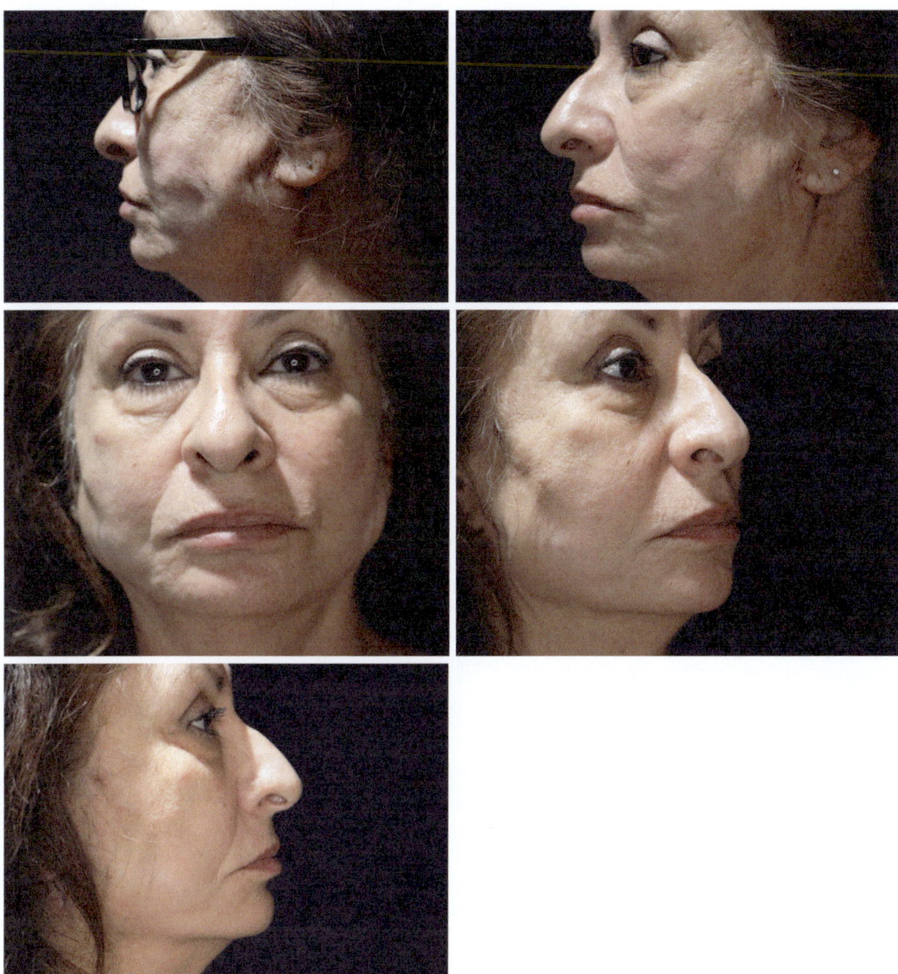

Figs. 33.27–33.31 Patient #2 immediately after the thread procedures

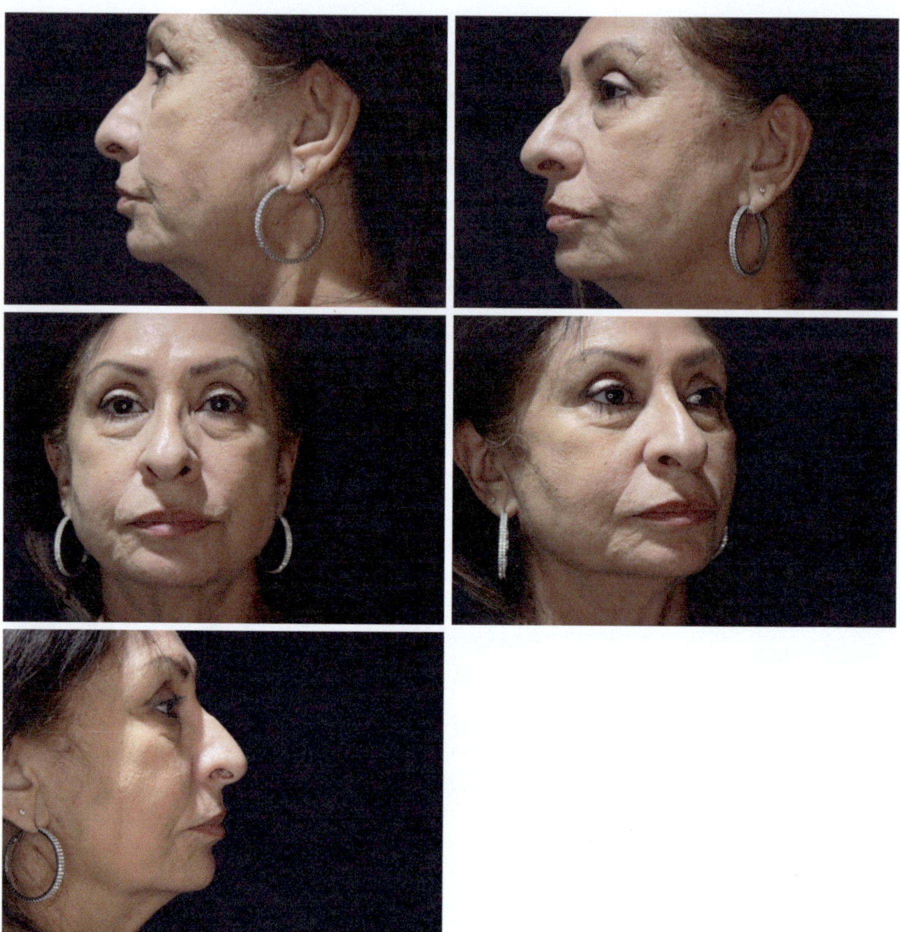

Figs. 33.32–33.36   Patient #2 at 2 weeks after the thread procedures

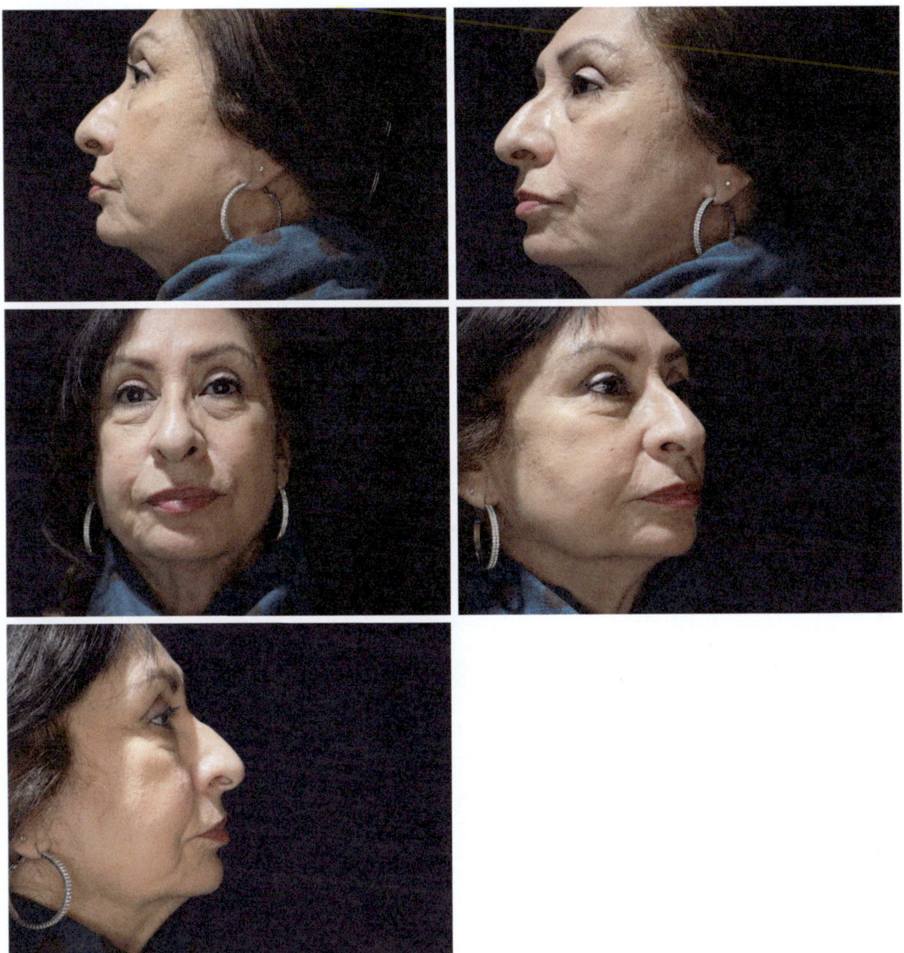

Figs. 33.37–33.41 Patient #2 at 1 month after the thread procedures

33.3 Patient #3

This patient although would benefit from a barbed thread lift of cheeks and jowls, was fearful of the barbed thread lift and was only willing to be treated with mesh threads. Thus, this patient is a good example of what areas can be treated with mesh threads as an alternative to gain improvement in skin quality.

This patient was treated with the following threads:

- 19 G × 38 mm mesh Boost threads × 4 for undereye region
- 19 G × 60 mm mesh Boost threads × 4 for crepey skin on lateral upper cheeks
- 19 G × 38 mm mesh Boost threads × 4 for nasolabial folds
- 19 G × 60 mm mesh Boost threads × 6 for chin and marionettes region

The lines drawn for the planned patterns of insertions are shown in Figs. 33.42, 33.43, and 33.44.

Figures 33.45 and 33.46 demonstrate the immediate appearance after the procedure. As one can see, the downtime for mesh threads would be much less than the barbed threads. There are only the small holes created for the thread insertions with no dimpling or buckling as can occur with barbed threads. There is also no need for any activity restrictions as there are with barbed threads. Discomfort is milder and resolves over several days.

Figures 33.47 and 33.48 show the patient's appearance before the procedure and her appearance 1 month afterwards. Although changes are not as dramatic as with barbed thread lift in photographs, there is significant improvement in skin quality that is appreciable by the patient.

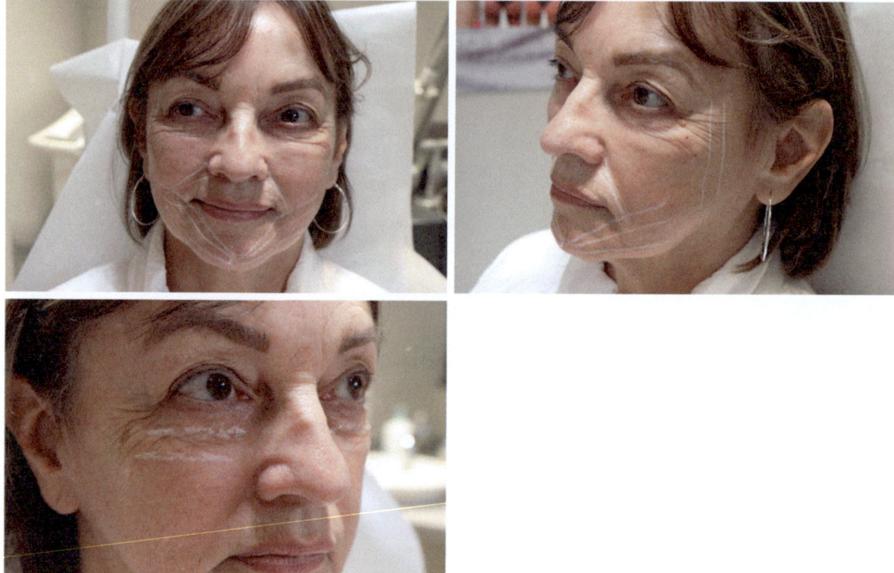

Figs. 33.42–33.44 Lines drawn for planned pattern of mesh thread insertions for patient #3

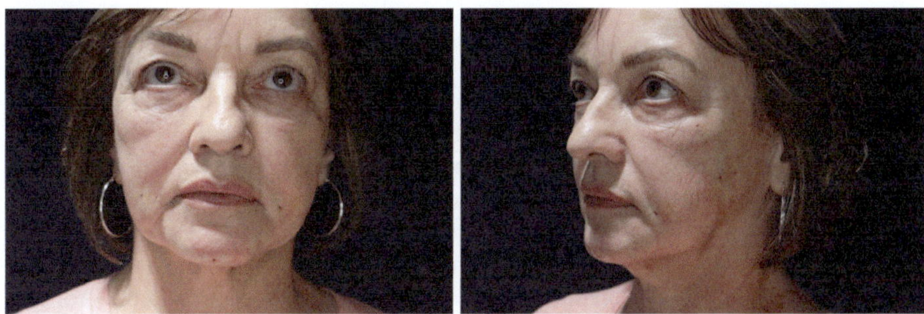

Figs. 33.45 and 33.46 Skin appearance immediately after thread insertions for patient #3

Fig. 33.47 Patient #3 before mesh thread procedures

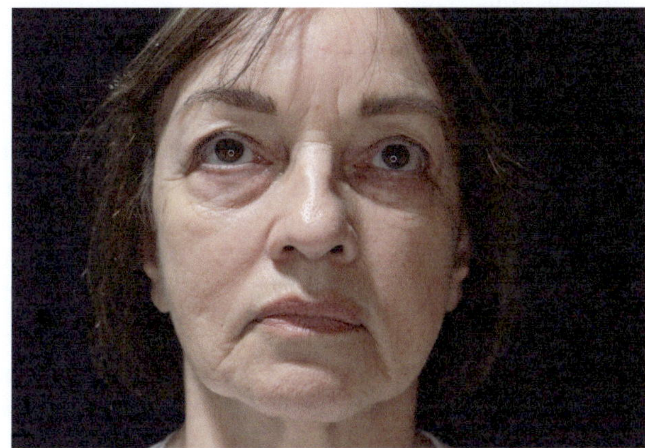

Fig. 33.48 Patient #3 1 month after mesh thread procedure

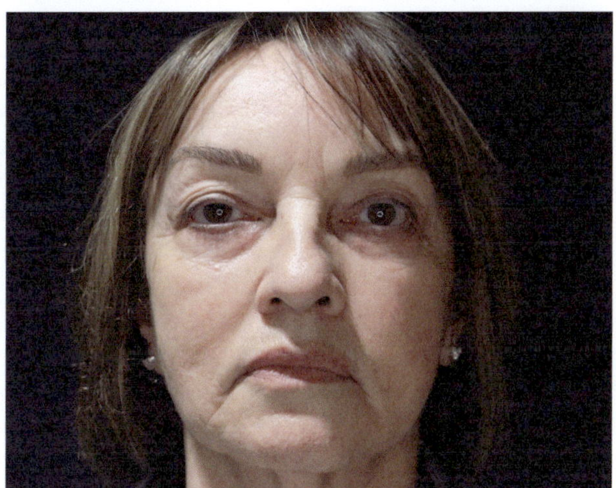

Appendix

This book is meant to be a primer for learning how to perform thread procedures. This book alone should not be utilized to begin performing thread procedures. It is still very important to observe the procedure and to have guided hands-on training. The next step in the process of learning how to perform thread procedures includes watching the instructional video included with this textbook. The instructional video demonstrates multiple thread procedures performed on a single patient during one visit. The procedures performed in the video include the most helpful for and most in demand by patients. These include thread lift of the cheeks, jowls, and neck with barbed threads and mesh thread procedures for undereye and nasolabial folds. The video is divided into three parts.

Instructional Video:

- **Part 1:** Demonstrates the preparation including the drawing of the patterns of thread placement to be performed.
- **Part 2:** Includes a demonstration of the local anesthesia injections and then the thread insertions for all of the procedures including thread lift of cheeks, jowls, and neck with barbed threads, mesh thread treatment of nasolabial folds and undereye regions.
- **Part 3:** Shows the final steps after thread insertion including assessment of results, adjustments of the threads to avoid dimpling, and then the cutting of the thread ends.

Watching this video will be very helpful in preparation for hands-on training. When seeking hands-on training, the source listed below is recommended since the thread names and types of procedures will match those described in this textbook.

Threads Supply and Training: Resculpt Medical Threads™
www.ResculptThreads.com
1-(888)-343-3383
sales@ResculptMedical.com
11500 West Olympic Blvd
Suite #525
Los Angeles, CA 90064

Index

© The Editor(s) (if applicable) and The Author(s), under exclusive license to
Springer Nature Switzerland AG 2023
N. M. Kim, *Non-Surgical Thread Procedures*,
https://doi.org/10.1007/978-3-031-36468-6

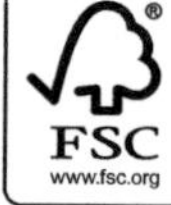

If you have any concerns about our products,
you can contact us on
ProductSafety@springernature.com

In case Publisher is established outside the EU,
the EU authorized representative is:
Springer Nature Customer Service Center GmbH
Europaplatz 3, 69115 Heidelberg, Germany

Printed by Libri Plureos GmbH
in Hamburg, Germany